Women Empowerment
and Role of Women Police

Women Empowerment and Role of Women Police

Edited by

Partha Pratim Sengupta
Anil Bhuimali
Sanjib Mandal
Sarmistha Bhattacharya
Bhupal Bhattacharya

CWP

Central West Publishing

Disclaimer
Every effort has been made by the publisher, editor and authors while preparing this book, however, no warranties are made regarding the accuracy and completeness of the content. The publisher, editor and authors disclaim without any limitation all warranties as well as any implied warranties about sales, along with fitness of the content for a particular purpose. Citation of any website and other information sources does not mean any endorsement from the publisher and authors. For ascertaining the suitability of the contents contained herein for a particular lab or commercial use, consultation with the subject expert is needed. In addition, while using the information and methods contained herein, the practitioners and researchers need to be mindful for their own safety, along with the safety of others, including the professional parties and premises for whom they have professional responsibility. To the fullest extent of law, the publisher, editor and authors are not liable in all circumstances (special, incidental, and consequential) for any injury and/or damage to persons and property, along with any potential loss of profit and other commercial damages due to the use of any methods, products, guidelines, procedures contained in the material herein.

A catalogue record for this book is available from the National Library of Australia

ISBN (print): 978-1-922617-07-1

About the Editors

Prof. Partha Pratim Sengupta is Professor of Economics and Head at the Department of Humanities and Social Sciences, National Institute of Technology Durgapur, India. He has been teaching at the institute for thirty-five years, out of which twenty years were devoted to teaching at PG level and research. More than twenty students have been awarded doctorate degree under the supervision of Prof. Sengupta. He has published more than one hundred research papers in national and international peer reviewed journals. He has been invited to deliver lectures at several conferences in India and abroad. He has also contributed chapters to edited volumes and has received several national and international academic awards. His areas of research interest include international economics, business economics, development economics and entrepreneurship management.

Prof. Anil Bhuimali, Ph.D., D.Litt., D.S.A., is the first Vice-Chancellor of Raiganj University, West Bengal, India and a former Professor of Economics, University of North Bengal, West Bengal, India. Born in a very small and poverty-stricken village in South Dinajpur of West Bengal and overcoming all hurdles in life, Prof. Bhuimali is an excellent academician of international repute today. He has taught and lectured at universities and institutes all over India and different countries across the globe. Prof. Bhuimali has to his credit over 50 monographs and edited-compilations and around 150 research-essays/articles. His areas of concentration are microeconomics, gender economics, international economics, rural economics, Dalit studies, Gandhian economics, development economics, IT policies & management, etc. Due to his profound eagerness in social-reforming, Prof. Bhuimali is presently involved in diverse humanitarian projects throughout West Bengal as well as India. He is a winner of several international and national awards. He was conferred the prestigious 'Banga Ratna Award' in 2016 by Government of West Bengal, India.

Sarmistha Bhattacharya is presently associated in the capacity of Assistant Professor at Department of Social Work, Law College Durgapur, India. She has around 7 years of teaching and administrative experience, besides 3 years of industrial experience. She has published scholarly articles in many prominent national and international journals and has edited two book volumes. She has obtained her BA, LL.B., MSW and is at the last phase of her Ph.D. from NIT Durgapur, India.

Dr. Sanjib Mandal is presently associated with the Department of Economics, Raiganj University, India in the capacity of Associate Professor. He is in active teaching profession for last two decades. He has executed administrative responsibility as Head of the Department of Economics at Sikkim Government College, Gangtok, India for more than a decade and has also acted as Chairman/Member of various Administrative/Technical Committees of Raiganj University. He has published a number of research papers and articles in various books and journals of repute. Dr. Mandal has been actively supervising M.Phil. and Ph.D. scholars at Department of Economics, Raiganj University. He was a member of Board of State Level Advisory Committee, MSME-DI Gangtok, Sikkim from 2012 to 2013. He has also functioned as a Coordinator of ASER (Annual Status of Education Report) Centre for the East District of Sikkim from 2009 to 2014 for ASER Study conducted in India. Dr. Mandal has also acted as an Editor of Annual Report (2018-19) of Raiganj University. He has participated in various national and international seminars, conferences and workshops. His areas of special interests include development economics, applied econometrics and policy research.

Dr. Bhupal Bhattacharya is presently associated with Department of Law, Raiganj University, West Bengal, India as an Assistant Professor. He has around 10 years of academic experience in different institutions including QS Ranked Banasthali Vidyapith (Deemed to be University) as an Associate Professor, Amity University Kolkata as Assistant Professor-III, Amity University Mumbai as Assistant Professor-II, NIT Durgapur as Adjunct Faculty and Law College Durgapur as Assistant Professor, in addition to 3 years of industrial and court experience. His academic qualifications include Ph.D. in Law, LL.M, MSW and B.Com (Hons.). He is in the editorial boards of many international and national journals. He has to his credit four edited books and one authored textbook on direct and indirect taxes, along with 37 scholarly research articles published in highly acclaimed international and national journals. He has chaired many international and national conferences and has also been invited as keynote speaker in many events.

Contents

Preface

A focus on the role of women in countries, especially in crisis and post-crisis situations, is very much needed while reviewing the progress toward gender equality and women's empowerment. The ongoing financial and economic crisis has also sparked widespread concern about its effect on such development goals.

Inspite of the growing recognition both nationally and internationally, women and girls continue to face discrimination based on their gender. An immediate action is needed to strengthen political commitment to reform the discriminatory laws and policies which have existed for generations. The women's efforts at home and at work are critical for enhancing food security and community resilience. The inclusion of women in the police force aims to strike a balance between providing safety and law enforcement while still safeguarding people's civil rights and liberties.

Most of the early literature on policing, including textbooks, are based on police administration highlighting the issues of the 1950s, 1960s, and 1970s. However, the field's focus has changed since then. The reformers are now focused on racial profiling, community relations, police discretion and use of force by police, among other concerns. Today's police conduct is better controlled than in the past, particularly since women began joining the force. More than ever before, police departments have become more diverse and inclusive.

This book focuses on the various aspects associated with women empowerment and role of women police. The efforts made by the governments and constitutional bodies towards achieving the goal of women empowerment have been highlighted, in Indian perspective.

List of Contributors

Vedant Saraf
Amity Law School (governed by Bar Council of India),
Kolkata, India

Jyoti Puri
Amity Law School (governed by Bar Council of India),
Kolkata, India

Aditi Daga
Faculty of Law,
Banasthali Vidyapith, Rajasthan, India

Sunidhi Sah
Faculty of Law,
Banasthali Vidyapith, Rajasthan, India

Sakshi Soni
Jamnalal Bajaj School of Legal Studies,
Banasthali Vidyapith, Rajasthan, India

Prachi Mishra
Jamnalal Bajaj School of Legal Studies,
Banasthali Vidyapith, Rajasthan, India

Purnima Sharma
Himachal Pradesh National Law University,
Shimla, India

Shreem Bajpai
Himachal Pradesh National Law University,
Shimla, India

Jatinder Singh
Department of Economics,
University of Jammu and Kashmir, India

Sujit Samanta
Additional District Inspector of Schools (Secondary Education)
Purba Burdwan, West Bengal, India

Rima Ghosh
Centre for Regulatory Studies, Governance and Public Policy, India

Santanu Panda
Centre for Regulatory Studies, Governance and Public Policy, India

Nancy Prasanna Joseph
SRM Institute of Science and Technology, Kattankulathur,
Tamilnadu, India

Abhishek Rajesh Bhattacharjee
Amity Law School,
Amity University, Kolkata, India

Shreya Das
Amity Law School,
Amity University, Kolkata, India

Subesha Banerjee
Law College Durgapur,
West Bengal, India

Sarmistha Bhattacharya
Department of Social Work,
Law College Durgapur
West Bengal, India

Anil Bhuimali
Raiganj University
West Bengal, India

Sanjib Mandal
Department of Economics,
Raiganj University,
West Bengal, India

Shivang Rawat
Amity Law School,
Amity University, Mumbai,
Maharashtra, India

Priyanka Shekhar
Banasthali Vidyapith,
Rajasthan, India

Vaishnavi Agarwal
Jamnalal Bajaj School of Legal Studies,
Banasthali Vidyapith,
Rajasthan, India

Sohini Das
Department of Social Work,
Law College Durgapur,
West Bengal, India

Email Jaison
Amity Law School,
Amity University, Mumbai,
Maharashtra, India

Muskan Jain
Jamnalal Bajaj School of Legal Studies,
Banasthali Vidyapith,
Rajasthan, India

Shibashish Bhattacharjee
Amity Law School,
Amity University, Kolkata,
West Bengal, India

Ankita Sen
Amity Law School,
Amity University, Kolkata,
West Bengal, India

Bhupal Bhattacharya
Raiganj University,
West Bengal, India

Sadaf Moosa
Haldia Law College,
West Bengal, India

1

Women Policing and Empowerment: Empowered, Yet in a Straitjacket of Gender Inequality

Vedant Saraf
Jyoti Puri

Abstract

Equality is the bastion of democracy and rule of law. Empowerment is a dynamic term that has seen a gradual yet effective change over the years. In the 17th century, the term empowerment was used to connote authority, vesting of power, to enable, etc., but in the later years, it became a password for women enablement and started encompassing the various aspects such as their social, economic, educational, political and psychological relation. Empowerment consequently leads to equal opportunities. In this study, our focus through the feminist lens would be based on the authority and its subsequent dissemination which gears the absence or presence of decision-making ability and proactive actions. To secure gender equality and dilute, if not eradicate, the existing disparity, it is not only enough to empower women, but invest in them the authority to make decisions and disseminate empowerment and enable others around them.

Introduction

The image of women has always been that of the weaker sex who needs to be protected. In such a stereotyped scene, being a policewoman in an entirely male-dominated masochistic is not an easy job. It is a general perception that policing requires one to be hardy, resilient, work at odd hours, and face situations wherein show of physical strength is paramount. Hence, women police, though being given the opportunity to work along with menfolk, are assigned to safer desk jobs with less stressful situations. Their work is generally restricted to assist the policemen when a woman convict is involved and not be given an independent role. Equality is the bastion of democracy and rule of law. As a citizen of a democratic country with an enriched and comprehensive Constitution, it is a given that there will be equal opportunities amongst men and women. Gender equality is the core of our preamble and is then enshrined in the fundamental rights and duties as well as Directive Principles of State policy. Equal Remuneration Act, 1976, among other Indian Government initiatives, was enacted to effectively curb gender discrimination and provide equal opportunities in recruitments and promotions. In reality, professionalism and feminism work against each other. Gender divisive roles have led to inequality though the opportunity exists.

Women in police fulfil stereotypical jobs, such as guarding young offenders and women inmates. In a technologically advanced world, women have gained from the internet in the field of their profession, expressing themselves and from networking. In doing so, their digital footprints have been misused by miscreants of the digital world to troll, hack, morph, bully, cyberstalk, defame, blackmail them, and also sometimes use pornographic images to intimidate, control, and cause tremendous mental torture. The perpetrators are difficult to identify, and this allows them to carry on their misadventure with impunity. It is natural that in cyber-related crimes, the contents may be too sensitive for the women to openly divulge the contents to any male police officer. Thus, many cases go unreported for the lack of women police being given the work of policing in such fields. In other cases of violence against women like rape, domestic violence, acid attacks, sexual harassment at the workplace, cases are seldom registered in the legal system and women generally avoid pursuing such cases.

The existence of equal opportunities will be the dipstick in the multi-layered social process of empowerment of women in police wherein it will be seen whether she has the capacity and equal opportunity to effectively put in use the power invested in her.

Whenever the image of police personnel comes to mind of any person, it is generally that of a male. Even though there is a steady increase in the women police personnel, they are still being underutilized. Nevertheless Natrajan (1996) feels that women officers have demonstrated their capability in performing various police tasks and are slowly finding their niche in this male-dominated occupation. With globalisation and the advancement of society, the rise in crime rates against women has also increased. In such a scenario, there is a necessity of an increase in women police personnel. Also, there is a need to give them equal powers like their counterparts to deal with women-oriented cases independently. Women, however, are slowly and steadily approaching this male-dominated field out of necessity and widening scope (Krishnamurthi, 1996).

The Need for Women Police in India

India's population consists of 45% women, but the literacy rate is 64.6% while the literacy rate for men is 80.9%. Indian women suffer not only discrimination but also poverty and ignorance. A number of laws have been enacted for women protection in India.

During British India, on 22nd November 1918, Mrs. Stanley was appointed as the first women Superintendent of police. With her appointment, an order was passed which suggested that 100 female police officers were to be directed by 10 superior officers. An order following this was issued after some time, specifying certain guidelines and qualifications for enrolment. Although this indicated a new ray of hope for women but there were certain criteria which again showed that women faced discrimination. The criteria which proved discrimination were:

- Women having dependent children were barred from service.
- Women were not to be sworn in as constables.
- Women were denied their right to a pension.

There were no such criteria that men had to face when enrolling themselves in the line of police work. The order passed above resulted in the appointment of 25 women police officers by 17th February 1919. Lilian Wyle, a renowned policewoman appointed among these 25 candidates, proved herself when she was awarded the British Empire Medal in 1949. She retired as an inspector. Although women proved themselves more than capable by their outstanding service in the first world war, all this soon came to an end. The economic crisis faced by the British after the first world war resulted in cuts in public expenditure. Since the women were not given the post of constables, their work did not come under the term "proper police work". This resulted in the abolition of the women police. In the year 1939, we again saw people in favour of women police because of their contributions during the first world war. Although women were being appointed as police, they still received low wages, and they were confined to one unit in particular and were mostly given clerical, juvenile, or guard duty work. They were hardly promoted and the promotions that took place were within their own women's unit. They were never promoted to perform basic patrol responsibilities, because of the male administration denying women of the experience they need. When federal law made it mandatory to give equal opportunities to everyone regardless of their gender or race, women could finally show their potential for police work.

The growing violence against women is proof of the lack of strictness in the legal system. The system over commits and under delivers. Cases of violence against women are hardly registered, and women are unwilling to pursue the case because of gender-based discrimination. The behaviour of the police along with the supporting legal civil-servants is disheartening. Women are unwilling to go to male police to report a crime. In order to avoid fear and disgrace, women do not register complaints against crimes like rape, domestic violence, etc. Crimes like harassment, stalking, domestic violence, are being committed all over the country but they are not reported because the victim might not be comfortable talking to a male police officer about it. The trauma of going through the incident once again, narrating the entire incident in front of a male police officer is one of the main reasons for the crime going unnoticed.

There are certain requirements that need to be fulfilled for the arrest and detention of women as well as for dealing with women victims. The law says that in order to search a women or in order to detain a women, a female police officer needs to be present, and this search cannot be performed by a male police officer. However, due to gender discrimination in the police force, there aren't enough women police officers. There is also a prejudiced attitude and behaviour within the police stations. Only a small percentage of the women population of the country is in the police force.

Among many other regulatory bodies, India's police's basic physical and organisational structures and facilities are imperfect. They generally lack proper training equipment. The police force has also carried certain successful operations, but that doesn't happen every time. The main reason for this is the government's tenacious catastrophe for investing in law implementation reforms and unwillingness for the development of infrastructure. The police sector has never been given the top priority since its initiation in 1947. The police force has proved their potential a number of times, but due to lack of infrastructure and lack of proper incentives by the authorities the desired results are not achieved every time.

In the year 1990, the government of Tamil Nadu took a decision of introducing All Women Police Units (AWPUs) for dealing with crimes against women such as rape, dowry deaths, etc. It was a thoughtful solution to the problem of crimes going unregistered due to the lack of women police. No doubt that the presence of these units of women officers would help women victims of domestic violence, rape, harassment, etc. A study was conducted in 2005 that yielded two benefits. They are as follows:

- Victims felt much more comfortable opening up to a female officer instead of a male officer, and
- Involvement of women police officers helped in the reduction of domestic abuse and brutality.

The studies in 1996, 2001, 2002 showed that these women officers were not professionally trained. Some officers found it difficult to help the victims because of a lack of judgement and due to a shortage of psychologists. The study yielded improvements in certain fields. They are as follows:

- Dispute resolution
- Interview techniques
- Data entry
- Date management.

If these problems were looked into the women officers would perform their duties efficiently.

Another major issue that comes to light is police brutality. Starting from the time of British India, on 13 April 1919, the Jallianwala Bagh massacre took place where a minimum of 400-500 people were murdered and many were injured due to the brutality by the police. In 2006, the police opened fire on people who were revolting and protesting against land acquisition for SEZ of Videocon. In 2019, the police thrashed students who were protesting at the campus of Jamia Milia Islamia. In 2020, the custodial death of a father son duo, who were beaten to death by policemen, shook the nation. In all these incidents, we see the result of police brutality by male policemen. Nowhere in these incidents, we see the names of women police because they would not resolve the issue by using such physical violence and cruelty.

Over time, we see that women are now recruited into departments of anti-terrorism, traffic police, and patrolling. Despite repeated efforts for the employment of women police officers and establishment of more All Women Police Units (AWPUs), the percentage is very low as compared to men police. A request has been made to the respective police departments for active women police and their position in respective departments. No matter what the situation, women police have performed their professional duties with utmost sincerity and are trying to restore the good name of the police department.

We have to blame ourselves for creating that macho image of police in the minds of the people in the society. Even in today's time women have to deal with societal restrictions and that manly image when adopting this as a profession. In order to choose this as a profession, the first and foremost step is to try and change the perception of society. Many appointed organizations are creating awareness for women to join the police department, informing us about the need for gender-based changes in the department.

Problems Faced by Women Police at Work and Home

The most important issue in the 21st century is work-life stability. Family and work go hand in hand. It's like two sides of the same coin. They both interfere with one another. As soon as the demand for one side increases, it leads to conflicts on the other side., leading to an imbalance.

Late working hours are a major problem faced by women police. There is a shortage of women police required in the department, thus, resulting in late working hours of existing employees. As already discussed above, the police departments are lacking proper infrastructure and incentives. The employees are paid less, and the working environment leads to a lack of motivation resulting in poor work performance. The excess workload is again a problem due to a lack of the required number of employees. The burden is given to existing employees to cover the work due to a lack of manpower. Sexual harassment is a problem that many women face. They are mistreated by people in the department itself. Long travel to work and lack of proper transport facility is another problem faced by many women police. The majority of police stations in the cities lack even the basic facilities such as sweepers, backup power, drinking water, and cooks, thus, greatly inconveniencing the staff. Gender discrimination is also a major issue that women have to deal with. They are denied equal opportunities and promotions because of their gender. Sometimes they are even exploited by higher authorities. Lack of coordination with other employees is again a major problem faced by women police on a day-to-day basis. Health issues are also one of the major issues faced by women at work. Being a police officer is a tiring job and there is a general perception that a man's physical strength is greater than that of a woman's strength. The health issues in women police lead to the job stress, thus, resulting in easy burnout. As the male-dominated society is not very welcoming to a female police officer, it may take her a long time to get adapted to the surroundings. Lack of proper training programs is again a major issue that a woman police officer faces. This leads to a lack of judgement and an inability to help a victim on many occasions.

A woman police officer has to face problems not only at work but also at her home. Suspicion by family members and society is a major problem. Even in the 21st century, a working and an independent woman faces such troubles. This is a problem that exists because of the mentality of the society. Late working hours, excess workload, and night shift hamper the family relationships, thus, causing disputes amongst the family members. Thus, it becomes difficult to carry out the responsibilities as a mother/wife/daughter because of these issues. The women in police do not get time for themselves and family. They cannot participate in any social and religious gatherings. Excessive workload and family pressure lead to a lack of time for personal grooming. Tension and challenges lead to health issues resulting in stress. Even after going through so much trouble, they are not compensated fairly. The promotions are generally denied because of gender, thus, the lack of incentives and low salary demotivate them day by day.

Solution to the Problems Faced by Women Police

Women face an infinite number of problems both on and off duty. This leads to a lack of will to work. The first solution to their problem is to create an equal balance by the higher authorities. The second solution to their problems is the sufficient budget. This would lead to the arrangement of proper transportation facilities and the development of the work environment and infrastructure for them. The third solution is the recruitment of new employees. Recruitment of willing candidates will result in proper distribution of work and would reduce the long working hours of the employees which would ultimately result in proper time management in every sphere of life. The fourth solution to their problems is less interference by the male senior members of the departments and proper coordination between the colleagues. Last but not least proper training facilities are required for women police. This would also mean proper physical and necessary military training for women police to deal with difficult situations with ease. Providing every woman police training in the technological departments and for crowd control would be immensely beneficial. Providing women with proper maternity leaves and flexible working hours will also help in increasing in workplace efficiency. These measures would result in a reduction of stress and better work-life balance for the women police. If the above measures are kept in mind and are implemented in due time, it will result in an improvement of the efficiency of women police and would encourage more women candidates to be employed at police departments.

Conclusion

The first police officer ever appointed was Alice Stebbins Wells, appointed in 1910 in Los Angeles. Thus, we can see that women have been engaged in the enterprise of policing for more than 110 years. It is noted that the condition of equality is enhancing, but at a slower pace. We can easily see that the work of women is being constrained by societal pressure and due to inequalities in every phase of life. Policewomen not only face problems and discrimination at work but also at their homes.

Being a police officer in a department while being a parent is different for male and female police officers. Disputes between work and home are generally seen for women police rather than male police. Studies conducted by different researchers often had the same result that women police are not given full authority over anything in the department because we are still living in a male-dominated society. Many studies show that women have been held back in attaining rank and file due to gender discrimination.

In 1994, 50 employees were interviewed regarding less number of women in the police department. Harassment was one of the main causes of the less number of women police. However, it was not the most important cause. The most important cause that came to light was the maternity leave. Due to a lack of provision dealing with maternity leave issues, women were being held back. Lack of flexible working hours, no extended career breaks, etc., were the issues they would eventually have to face if they had or ever wanted a family.

Promotion and greater opportunities in the career are thought to be provided equally, however, in reality, it is many times determined by the gender. Discrimination leads to unequal opportunities. Police work is still considered a male-dominated field that requires physical strength. The overall masculine image makes it harder for the women police personnel to get cases relating to crime against women, as it is thought that it is not possible for them to take on the mantle of saviours. The increasing crime rate against women can be best handled by the women police personnel as the victims being women would feel free to come up to women for redressal of their grievances. Thus, the women serving in the police force need to be given equal status and opportunity in the workforce like their male counterparts not only as a measure of empowering them in the right sense but also to facilitate victims by empowering them to come forward without any fear of the protector turning into a predator.

If there is an increase in the number of policewomen at all stages, it will certainly result in a significant change in the cultural heritage of the society for the greater good.

References

Natarajan, M. (1989). Towards Equality: Women Police in India. *Women & Criminal Justice, 8(2)*, 1-18.

Krishnamurthi, L. (1996). Role Conflicts and Tension of Women Police. *The Indian Journal of Social Work, 57(4),* 615-629.

Carol Martin (1996). The impact of equal opportunities policies on the day-to-day experiences of women police constables. *British Journal of Criminology, 36(4),* 510-528.

Simon Holdaway and Sharon K. Parker (1998). Policing Women Police. *British Journal of Criminology, 38(1),* 40-60.

Jennifer M. Brown (1998). Aspects of Discriminatory Treatment of women police officers serving in forces in England and Whales. *British Journal of Criminology, 38(2),* 265-282.

Mangai Natarajan (2006). Dealing with domestic disputes/violence by women police in India: Results of a training program in Tamil Nadu. *International Journal of Criminal Justice Sciences, 1(1),* 1-19.

Cara E. Rabe-Hemp (2009). POLICEwomen or PoliceWOMEN?: Doing Gender and Police Work. *Feminist Criminology, 4(2),* 114-129. https://doi.org/10.1177/1557085108327659

Zaigham Sarfraz and Asma Naureen (2016). Empowering Women: A Case of Women Police Force in Pakistan. *Lyallpur Historical & Cultural Research Journal, 2(1),* 13-27.

2

Role of Women Policing in Relation to Forced Prostitution and Trafficking

Vaishnavi Agarwal

Abstract

Trafficking is a serious offence which involves a series of acts. Till now, no reliable or exact data of trafficked women and girl children is available. Trafficking is the root cause of forced prostitution. Forced prostitution is the source of earning gains for the unscrupulous sections of the society. Sometimes, due to poverty, the parents sell their children, but they forget about the dreams of their offsprings. The other aspects of trafficking involve forcing the women as house servant, beggars, etc. The women and girls who suffer from trafficking become victims in the eyes of the society, however, they are truly never accepted by the society. The rate of crime reporting is also very low. Further, the victims are sadly seen with suspicion if the police catches them.

Major steps are needed to be taken to prevent the trafficking and forced prostitution. NHRC has launched numerous actions on trafficking with the involvement of the Department of Women and Child Development, Government of India. Due to these initiatives, many victims have been rescued.

Introduction

The word prostitution refers to a practice of sexual activity in return of money or any other kind of benefit. The legal status of prostitution varies from country to country and even sometimes region to region. In India, it is illegal. Some enter into this business by their will or desire, whatsoever is the reason behind it. However, forcing women in this activity against their wish on the orders of their master becomes forced prostitution. It represents a gross exploitation of the rights of women and girl children. Thus, the females in the society are occasionally treated as an object. However, this perception can be changed by revolution and awakening.

Human trafficking is an organised series of crime which occur at different places at different times. The main crime involved in human trafficking is the transfer, exploitation and commercialisation of human beings. Human trafficking is a never ending process of crime as it does not stop at selling or transferring women and girl children. The various objectives of trafficking of people may be labour, begging, slavery, prostitution, escort services and so on. Sadly, the portrayal of the word 'SHE' as miserable, weak, object, etc., has continued from the old times.

"Trafficking in persons as the recruitment, transportation, transfer, harbouring or receipt of persons, by means of threat or use of force or other forms of coercion, abduction, fraud, deception, abuse of power or position of vulnerability or giving or receiving of payments or benefits to achieve the consent of a person having control over another person, for the purpose of exploitation"[1]. Exploitation shall include, at a minimum, prostitution, forced labour or services, slavery or practices similar to slavery, servitude or the removal of organs.[2]

"The trafficking and forced prostitution of a woman and child is a very serious crime and abuse to the human rights of a person." The trafficking in women and children is increasing day by day, and it is very difficult to find out the exact numbers. At global level, a significant number of children and women disappear every year. Many of these incidents are not even registered due to many reasons.

Reasons

In today's scenario, trafficking is very common and happens in each part of the world. It can be present in different forms, however, it happens everywhere. The main reason for trafficking is to earn gains or money. To understand why the women and girl children are mostly targeted for trafficking and forced prostitution, it is necessary for us to understand its causes. The following are the reasons:

---

[1] United Nations General Assembly (2000). Protocol to Prevent, Suppress and Punish Trafficking in Persons Especially Women and Children, supplementing the United National Convention against Transnational Organized Crime. Article 3.
[2] UNODC. Available from http://www.unodc.org/unodc/en/human-trafficking/what-is-human-trafficking.html.

❖ Poverty: It is one of the main reasons for trafficking and forced prostitution of women and girl children. Many parents sell their children in exchange of money without thinking about the suffering of the children. This leads to total sacrifice of the dreams and innocence of the victims.

❖ Natural disasters: Any natural calamity leads to economic instability in that particular area. As a result, the people are not able to fulfil their basic needs. The traffickers take advantage of this opportunity to abduct girl children and women. Occasionally, these activities are also carried out in the guise of food or work.

❖ The large amounts of profit can be earned through these types of activities.

❖ Search for better life: Sometime the search for better life leads to the people on both sides of this social issue to indulge in such activities.

❖ Demand for cheap labour: There is need for the cheap labour in our society as industries and other manufacturers want to enhance their profit. Traffickers get profit from the supply of cheap labour for the work. There is also a demand for commercialized sex due to which traffickers get more opportunities to exploit women and girl children.

Consequences

Trafficking and forced prostitution leave a significant impact on the physical and mental well-being of millions of women and girl children in the world. The trauma which the victims suffer varies from victim to victim as it depends on circumstances and conditions in which they are kept. Some consequences generally suffered by the victims are mentioned below:

• They are displaced from the community. The people blame them for whatever happened to them, and they are treated badly by community. They are usually thrown out from their own houses on their return due to the so-called respect of family and society.

- They are isolated from their own environment, leading to mental issues.
- They do not get sufficient rest and sleep.
- Various health problems occur, like STDs, HIV, depression, trauma, etc.
- The women suffer from miscarriage and abortion.
- They are deprived of medical care and hygiene.
- Many children who had their kidneys removed by traffickers for organ sale face serious problems.
- They become psychologically/emotionally disturbed, with thoughts and feelings such as:
  o Helplessness and withdrawal
  o Dissociation
  o Self-blame and identification with aggressor
  o Distraction
  o Foreshortened view of time
  o Psychiatric disorders, including post-traumatic stress, depressive and eating disorders.

Legal Frameworks

❖ *International Conventions*

The Convention to Suppress the Slave Trade and Slavery of 1926:
Article (2) that the parties agreed "to prevent and suppress the slave trade "and to progressively bring about "the complete elimination of slavery in all its forms."

The Universal Declaration of Human Rights of 1948:
Article 4 of UDHR deals with slavery. It states that "no one shall be held in slavery or servitude; slavery and the slave trade shall be prohibited in all their forms."

The Covenant on Civil and Political Rights of 1966:
Article 8 states that "1. No one shall be held in slavery; slavery and the slave trade in all their forms shall be prohibited. 2. No one shall be held in servitude. 3. No one shall be required to perform forced or compulsory labour."

The Convention on the Elimination of All Forms of Discrimination against Women of 1979:

Article 6 mentions that states parties to can take all appropriate measures, including legislation, to suppress all forms of traffic in women and exploitation of prostitution of women."

The Convention on the Rights of the Child of 1989:
States parties must "take all appropriate national, bilateral and multilateral measures to prevent the abduction of, the sale of or traffic in children for any purpose or in any form"

The Convention on the Rights of All Migrant Workers and Members of their Families of 1990:
Article 11 provides that no migrant worker or member of his or her family shall be held in slavery or servitude and not required to perform forced or compulsory labour ".

The Hague Convention on Protection of Children and Cooperation in respect of Inter-Country Adoption of 1993:
It provides in Article 32 that "no one shall derive improper financial or other gain from an activity related to an inter-country adoption".

The Declaration on the Elimination of Violence against Women of 1993:
The Declaration defines "violence against women" to include "rape, sexual abuse, sexual harassment and intimidation at work, in educational institutions and elsewhere, trafficking in women and forced prostitution."

The Rome Statute of the International Criminal Court of 1998:
Article 7 "Crimes against Humanity "to include "Enslavement" which means "the exercise of any and all of the powers attaching to the right of ownership over a person, in particular women and children."

The Optional Protocol to the Convention on the Rights of the Child, on the Sale of Children, Child Prostitution, Child Pornography of 2000:
The Optional Protocol stipulates, in Article 10, that states parties to must "take all necessary steps to strengthen international cooperation by multinational, regional and bilateral agreements for the prevention, detection, investigation, prosecution and punishment of those responsible for acts involving the sale of children, child prostitution, child pornography and child sex tourism."

United Nation Convention on Transnational Organised Crime (UN-TOC) and its Protocol against Trafficking persons:

It is the convention which deals with the issue and problem of human trafficking in a global perspective. This came into force on 25th December 2003 and was adopted by General Assembly on 15th November 2000. This convention contains/includes three major components:

o List of activities that form part of trafficking.
o Means and methods used in trafficking.
o Purpose or intention behind trafficking.

The Protocol of Trafficking:

In this protocol, the states are bound to arrange all necessary instruments for taking preventive measures for protection of victim and an offensive against the criminal core of the business.

United Nations office of Drug and Crime:

It is to prohibit the human trafficking and to prevent the smuggling of migrants. It also has a voluntary trust fund for victims of human trafficking which provides legal, financial and humanitarian aid to victim through different medium.

❖ *Indian Laws Relating Trafficking and Child Prostitution*

The Constitution of India:

- Article 15(3) enables the state to make special provisions for woman and children even if they are discriminatory.
- Article 21 gives right to live life with dignity and also gives the personal liberty to the people.
- Article 23 deals with prohibition of trafficking in human beings, forced labour and all forms of exploitation. This was aimed at putting an end to all forms of trafficking in the human beings including prostitution and beggary.
- Article 39(e) deals with the health and strength of workers, men, women.
- Article 39(f) insists that children be given opportunities to develop in a healthy manner so that childhood and youth are protected.

These articles given in Constitution state that the women and children should be given protection and they have the right to live their life as they want.

The Indian Penal Code:

The Indian Penal Code lends a helping hand to the special laws enacted to curb prostitution by attacking the source of this evil. Section 366A makes procreation of a minor girl from one part of place to another punishable and section 366B makes importation of a girl below the age of 21 years punishable. Sections 372 (selling minor for purposes of prostitution) and 373 make selling and buying of minor girls for the purpose of prostitution a crime for which even 10 years of imprisonment and fine can be awarded.

Suppression of Immoral Traffic in Women and Girls Act, 1956:

Trafficking was first dealt with by the Suppression of Immoral Traffic in Woman and Girls Act, 1956, which was passed on 31st December, 1956. This act is aimed to rescue the exploited women and girls, to prevent deterioration of public morals and to stamp out the evil of prostitution rampant in some parts of the country. According to SITA, prostitution is not illegal per se. The prostitute can carry on her trade wherever she likes subject to certain restrictions.

The Criminal Procedure Code, 1973:

The Criminal Procedure Code of 1973 also protects girls from sexual exploitation. It states that a presiding Judge or District Magistrate may, upon complaint that a female child under the age of 18 years is abducted or unlawfully detained, order the immediate restoration of the girl to her liberty or to her parent, guardian or husband. Section 98 is intended to give immediate relief to a woman or girl abducted or detained for any unlawful purpose. An action under this section cannot be taken except upon complaint made on oath.

The Immoral Traffic Prevention Act 1986:

This Act provides greater punishment to persons who cause, aid or abet the seduction of women and girls, over whom they have authority or who are in their care and custody for prostitution. This Act empowers the central government to appoint trafficking officers. These special police officers can search without warrant any premises where this offence is suspected of being committed, and they can rescue any person who is being forced into prostitution or is carrying on or is being made to carry on prostitution.

Rescue and Rehabilitation of Children and Minors under the ITPA, 1986:

When a magistrate has reason to believe from information received from the police or from any other person authorized by the state government that any person is living on, or is being made to carry on prostitution in a brothel, he may direct a police officer not below the mark of sub-inspector to enter such brothel and to remove such person and produce the person before him.

Indecent Representation of Women (Prohibition) Act, 1986:
The object of the Act was to prohibit indecent representation of women through advertisements or in publications, writings, paintings, figures or in any other manner. It defines 'indecent representation of women' as the depiction in any manner of a figure of a woman, her form of body or any part thereof in such a way as to have the effect of being indecent, or derogatory to, or is likely to deprave, corrupt or injure public morality.

The Juvenile Justice (Care and Protection of Children) Act, 2000:
This Act has elaborates the provisions for the care, protection, treatment, education, vocational training, development and rehabilitation of children rescued from those procuring, inducing or taking person for the sake of prostitution and detaining person in premises where prostitution is carried on. The definition specifically includes the child who is found vulnerable and is, therefore, likely to be induced into trafficking.

The Trafficking of Persons (Prevention, Protection and Rehabilitation) Bill, 2018:
The Bill creates a law for investigation of all types of trafficking, and rescue, protection and rehabilitation of trafficked victims. The Bill provides for the establishment of investigation and rehabilitation authorities at the district, state and national level. Anti-trafficking units are to be established to rescue victims and investigate cases of trafficking. Rehabilitation committees are to be set up to provide care and rehabilitation to the rescued victims. The Bill classifies certain purposes of trafficking as 'aggravated' forms of trafficking. These include trafficking for forced labour, bearing children, begging, or for inducing early sexual maturity. Aggravated trafficking attracts a higher punishment. The Bill sets out penalties for several offences connected with trafficking. In most cases, the penalties set out are higher than the punishment provided under the prevailing laws.

End Child Prostitution and Trafficking-Ecpat International:
It is a non-governmental organization and a global network of civil society organization exclusively dedicated to ending the Commercial Sexual Exploitation of Children (CSEC). It focuses on ending four main manifestations of CSEC: child pornography, the exploitation of children in prostitution, the trafficking of children for sexual purposes and the sexual exploitation of children in travel and tourism.

Role of Women Policing

With reference to the earlier mentioned legal consequences, it seems that very strict laws and regulations govern our nation. However, it is wrong to say that mere laws can help to overcome this issue. The help of the police as well as community is vital to catch the offenders. Whenever any such incident takes place, the family must go to the nearby station to lodge the FIR of the missing girl. Subsequently, the police officer must take all the necessary action. The civil society organisations must also come forward to help the police and communities.

3

Dowry: The Burning Bride

Aditi Daga
Sunidhi Sah

"Any young man, who makes dowry a condition to marriage, discredits his education and his country and dishonors womanhood" - Mahatma Gandhi

Abstract

Marriage is considered to be a sacrosanct union of two bodies. It not only creates a pious relationship between two individuals but also among their respective families until this custom was twisted by the society for its pleasure to fulfill their materialism. That is how "Dakshana" which was done earlier during "Kanyadan" turned into a barter system that involved the exchange of bride in return for some articles be it money, movable or immovable property. The extravagant demands do not come to an end anytime soon and the female has to go through an endless cycle of insults, physical violence, and lifelong trauma. Numerous beloved daughters have lost their lives, however, the situation has not changed much even today. In this chapter, we discuss the origin of dowry, it's implication and where our laws are failing.

In this study, we have specifically focused on the meaning of dowry, dowry system in different religions, effects/impacts on society, prevailing criminal status of dowry, inability of the laws to curb the dowry deaths, and impact of television on the mindset of society.

Introduction: Meaning of Dowry

Since time immemorial, a woman has always been a symbol of power, kindness, motherhood, and love. In ancient times, women were treated with respect, however, with the passage of time, people molded the traditions and culture for their benefit. This greediness welcomed an increasing number of crimes in the society like child marriage, dowry, etc. It is ironic how crimes like female infanticide are committed just to avoid future dowry burdens without even realizing how woman is the source of life herself.

What is dowry? How can it be the reason for not wanting a girl child? Is dowry a tradition or a crime? Dowry is a kind of gift like property, cash, car, jewellery, etc., given by the bride's father to the bridegroom or to his family as one of the conditions of marriage. Basically, the money or property that the bride brings to the groom's house as a kind of entry fees. It is referred to as 'dahez' in some parts of India. Dowry represents more like a liability or burden on the bride's father. It creates a burden on the shoulder of the bride's father. Often, to fulfil the high demand, he has to take a loan at a high-interest rate or even has to sell own property. It has always been treated as a symbol of showing high prestige. Many times, the inability of the bride's family to provide the dowry leads to torture and abuse against the bride. It is believed by the people that a higher dowry would lead to a better treatment of the bride after the wedding, and she will enjoy all her life. However, in reality, dowry is like a drug. It is so addictive that the groom's family never gets satisfied out of it. In ancient times, the gifts never played a major role, as they were just treated as the gift and not the entry fees. However, nowadays, the mask of tradition is used as per their own convenience to commit these crimes against the women.

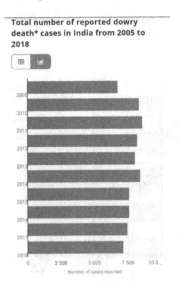

Source: Statista

Dowry and Religion

A religion represents a set of beliefs, thoughts, and practices. The religion is a guiding principle for numerous people in society and plays a major role in shaping the thinking and the way of living of a society. Therefore, it is important to understand what are the practices of dowry in these widely practiced religions around the world.

Christianity

Christians do not promote dowry nor they have completely put a stop on this practice. When Christians came to India, they did adopt various practices that inspired them. With time, the dowry system is becoming more prevalent in the Christian marriages, but cannot be regarded as rigid as other religions.

Islam

In Islam, marriage is regarded as a Nikah. It involves proposal, acceptance, consent, and other essential elements. Nikah makes the copulation legal and, thus, creates a relationship between the husband and wife. In terms of dowry, there is no such proficient practice of dowry, rather the opposite of dowry called dower (mehr) is followed in which the husband is bound to pay a certain amount to his wife either before marriage or after marriage. It is regarded as a mark of respect towards the wife and it also indicates the financial capacity of the husband in providing an admirable life to the wife. Dower can be in the form of some movable and immovable things, depending on the groom.

Hinduism

If we try to understand the dowry system in the Vedic Era, it is noted to be completely different from what dowry has turned in today's times. The Atharveda identifies various forms of marriage Divya, Prajapt, Arsha, etc. As the women during that period were not able to inherit property, hence dowry became a means to ensure that she has some belonging of her own. In the Braham form of marriage, the practice of gifting daughters was prevalent, however, this cannot be regarded as a dowry as it involved the father gifting articles voluntarily out of love and affection, and it presented no impediment in the settlement of the daughter's marriage. Another reason was to attract more number of the bridegroom and choose the most suited one for them.

Implications of Dowry

Dowry is a social evil of our society and its impact is not restricted to the sufferer (the woman) only, as it creates an endless cycle of agony and disturbance in the lives of her parents' family as well to such an extent that the birth of a girl is no more rejoiced. The following are a few major examples of what dowry practice leads to:

Gender Imparity

As per the report titled "Signs of Change: Sex Ratio Imbalance and Shifting Social Practices in Northern India" conducted by Mattis Laursen and Ravinder Kaur, a large disparity in the sex ratio in the northern cities of India mainly Kurukshetra (in Haryana), Kangra (Himachal Pradesh) and Fatehgarh Sahib (Punjab) has been observed.

		SC/ST	OBC	Other Castes	Total
Is there a shortage of brides in your community as a result of sex-selective abortions?	Yes	85 (37.6)	77 (48.1)	131 (52.6)	293 (46.1)
	No	141 (62.4)	83 (51.9)	118 (47.4)	342 (53.9)
Total		226	160	249	635

Percentages in parentheses.
Source: Data collected by authors.

The implications of dowry are deep-rooted. Since the birth of a girl child, it is believed that the girl has to be sent off to her husband's house, and to do so would require a good expense and undoubted heavy sum of money as dowry. This leads to a mindset of accumulation of wealth, which also hampers the growth of women. Thus, marriage is made as the sole objective of her life. She is regarded as a burden, which gives her a lifelong agony and a feeling of dislike and no belongingness.

Social Effects

A major chunk of the population resides in rural India where dowry is widely practiced. Therefore, every other family is a victim of this evil practice. A vicious cycle is created when one family demands dowry and the other family fulfils the demand. In the next turn, the family that once gave the dowry steps forward to further demand dowry for their son. This leads to an endless cycle of taking and giving dowry that does nothing except instigation of the feelings of greed, corruption, and hatred, where marriage does not remain a pious social affair.

Deterioration of the Dignity of Women

It is quite ironic that birth of a girl child especially in a country like India, where the goddess is worshiped in every part of the country, is considered as a bad omen. It is surprising how this poor status of women is not restricted to just villages but even in the cities where a big portion of well-educated people reside. A girl who is looked down upon since her birth till death faces the endless cycle of insult and backwardness, thus, hampering her educational, emotional, and mental growth. The continuous attempt to bring equality drastically fails on its face when a woman is regarded as inferior and unwanted gender as if they are nothing but just like cattle to be sold off and get away from the liability as early as possible.

Heinous Crime

According to the Times of India report (2016), a man in Jharkhand sold off his wife's kidney to fulfil his greed of dowry. Even after this, the wife was tortured and, in the end, she took her own life. This indicates how greed at times turns a person into nothing less than a demon. Several cases in India relate to domestic violence where the woman is badly beaten up for less dowry or nonfulfillment of the demands. This violence takes up a more aggravated form in which the women is even burnt alive. Dowry deaths seem like an ongoing cycle that has no end. A report by NCB indicates that up to 21 deaths per day were reported in the year 2016, not considering those deaths which are still to be investigated or are simply not reported by the families.

Trauma to the Bride's Family

The ordeal of dowry practice is not only restricted to the daughter, but it also puts the strain on the family to arrange dowry before marriage and to fulfil the other demands after marriage. There are ample examples in which the family of the bride had to sell off their assets to ensure a better life for their daughter just to find themselves at a financial crisis leading to either indebtedness or other mental issues. Needless to say, this social evil should be eradicated for the society and nation to achieve the real progress and development.

Loss of Self-esteem Among Women

The research titled "Terror as a Bargaining Instrument: A Case Study of Dowry Violence in Rural India" was conducted by Vijayaendra Rao and Francis Bloch (2013) in the villages of southern states of India. As observed, the women's family paying less dowry were subjected to violence. The wife had a pressure on her to further ensure giving birth to a male child only and was further disrespected for giving birth to a girl child. The open-ended interview clearly indicated that the husband was happier and more satisfied if the wife gave birth to a son. It is hard to imagine the plight of a woman who is regarded as a burden in her enter life time both by her family and subsequently by her in-laws. It is shocking that how the amount of respect a woman gets depends entirely on the amount of dowry she brings as if no other element in human life seems more valuable.

Criminal Status

DOWRY is dealt under the Indian Penal Code, Criminal Procedure Code, and Evidence Act

Women need a safe and carefree environment with all the respect that a man enjoys in the nation, therefore, dowry has given a status of crime in India. It cannot be demanded in the name of tradition. If found, guilty are to be punished and prosecuted under the respective law. Many laws have been passed since independence to prohibit the practice of dowry but the root cause of the problem is the Inheritance Laws. After Indian independence in 1947, the Hindu Succession Act was passed 1956 giving the right to women to inherit the ancestral property, but it did not bring objective equality between men and women in terms of inheritance. for example, married daughters had no residential right in the ancestral home.

Laws prohibiting dowry: **DOWRY PROHIBITION ACT ,1961 ; IPC SECTION 304B AND 498A; PROTECTION OF WOMEN FROM DOMESTIC VIOLENCE ACT, 2005 and many more**

The Dowry Prohibition Act 1961 states "dowry means any property or valuable security given or agreed to be given either directly or indirectly (a) by one party in a marriage to the other party in marriage; or (b) by the parents of either party to a marriage or by any other person to either party to a marriage or to any other persons at or before or after the marriage as consideration for the marriage of the said parties, but does not include dower or mehr in the case of persons to whom the Muslim Personal law applies.

Section 304B was inserted in the Indian Penal Code,1860 under which dowry death is a definite offense punishable with a minimum sentence of imprisonment for 7 years and maximum imprisonment for life. It states that if the death of women is caused by bodily injury or burns or occurs in suspicious circumstances within 7 years of her marriage, and there's evidence to show that before her death, she was subjected to cruelty or harassment by her husband or his relative regarding the demand for dowry, then the husband or the relative shall be deemed to have caused her death.

Section 113B of the Evidence Act, 1872, makes an extra presumption of dowry death when it is shown that before her death, the woman had been subjected to cruelty on account of dowry demand. Section 304B IPC along with Section 113B of the Evidence Act have enabled the conviction of many who were not caught by the Dowry Prohibition Act, 1961. **Section 113A** of the Evidence Act provides a similar presumption of abetment of suicide (which is an offense under **Section 306 IPC**), in case of death of a married woman within seven years of her marriage.

The judiciary additionally includes murder charges under **Section 302 IPC** as this allows courts to impose the death penalty on perpetrators of the offense. **Section 406 IPC**, pertaining to offenses for the criminal breach of trust, applies in cases of recovery of dowry as it is supposed to be for the benefit of the woman and her heirs.

Section **498A IPC** was specifically included in 1983 to protect women from cruelty and harassment. The constitutionality of Section 498A was challenged before the Supreme Court of India on grounds of abuse, on grounds that it gave arbitrary power to the police and the court. However, it was upheld in Sushil Kumar Sharma v. Union of India (2005). The Code of Criminal Procedure (1973) provides that for the prosecution of offenses under Section 498A IPC, the court can take cognizance only when it receives a report of the facts from the police or upon a complaint being made by the victim or her family.

Failure to Curb Dowry Deaths

Even though the effective laws have been formulated, however, the widespread dowry system is still not under control. Dowry which was earlier practiced in certain states of northern India among only certain castes of people is not restricted anymore and has gotten into even in rural areas of southern India. It is quite evident that there are certain lacunas in the laws. Following are some examples of such loopholes.

Ambiguous Terms in the Laws

As per the Dowry Prohibition Act (originally passed in 1961 and amended twice in the 1980s), dowry is defined as 'any property or valuable security given or agreed to be given either directly or indirectly by one party to a marriage to the other party to the marriage or by the parents of either party to a marriage or by any other person, to either party to the marriage or to any other person at or before [or any other time after the marriage] in connection with the marriage of the said parties. Here it is not clearly defined as to what articles would come under the preview of dowry. It is considered that giving voluntary gifts is not dowry but it is ignored that in the name of voluntary gifts, a significant pressure is on the bride's family to fulfil the insanely expensive dowry demands.

Lack of Proper Enforcement of Law and Low Prosecution Rate

Even considering the sensitivity of the cases involved in dowry death, the government had issued certain guidelines according to which investigation of such cases should be done. However, the police sometimes fails to implement these and they still stick to their traditional technique of investigation which is lengthy and usually not successful. In this era of scientific advancement, it is required that modern methods of an investigation involving forensic science should be used. In such cases, the dying declaration plays an extremely important role, and the police should ensure that they record the declaration in their own presence. Another important aspect is that the witness does not turn hostile and is neither silenced. Such cases require quick investigation and filing of charge sheet.

The data below indicates the imbalance between the reported cases and number of actual convictions, thus, indicating failures in putting an end to dowry and taking strict actions against the guilty.

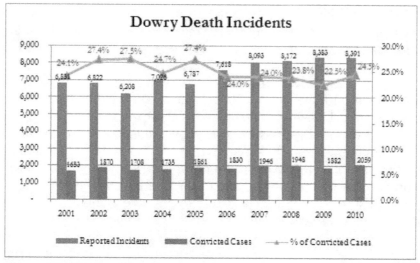

Source: World Press Bride Burning

Less Punishment to Dowry Givers

We cannot ignore the fact that dowry givers (the bride's family) at the time of marriage fulfil the demand of the groom's family without raising their voice against it. They are equally responsible for promoting the practice of dowry.

Societal Mindset

As long as society will keep treating women inferior, depriving them of their rights of getting proper education so that they could reach a position where they are independent enough to stand for themselves, such crimes will not end. We have to go deep into the rural areas where women are treated very badly. Unless the problem is not solved at the grassroots level, we cannot expect significant changes. The policies and plans by the government will be of no good unless they are properly implemented. Education gives a sense of courage to a woman to walk out of an abusive marriage and to exercise her right as a dignified strong woman.

Television and its Impact

Cinema is an influential medium of delivering and it gains the strength from the audience, i.e., us. The moving reel of pictures is nothing but the expression which is supposed to be felt by everyone watching it. There is hardly any section of society which has not seen any movie or any daily soap. Cinema is moving towards an increasing number of movies and daily soaps with some social issues like, "Matrubhoomi: A Nation Without Women", "English Vinglish", "Thappad", "Antardwand" (won the National Film Award for Best Film on social issues at the 2009 National Awards) and the list is never-ending. Likewise, the daily soaps also came forward to spread awareness about these issues. It is appreciable that some directors came out of the league to serve content that is not only entertaining but leaves a meaningful impact on both heart and mind, as Television is not only for entertainment purpose but also for the social cause. History is full of incidents as to how the media was able to bring a mass uproar and modification in the society.

Over the last three decades, there have been hundreds of serial dramas on-air on the Indian television, and these have become an important part of the day to day lives of the common people. These shows or movies have influenced a huge portion of society. Most of them left their essence to the core of the audience's heart. The mindset of the audience that the movies or dramas are for entertainment only has changed in the last one decade, and people are moving towards content with some serious issues, the audience is getting matured and demanding for better content than usual family soaps and comedies. Thus, the television medium is a lot more than just entertainment. We need to experience something deep that touches cords, something which we observe in daily lives but never got bothered about that. Therefore, these reels of pictures are a way necessary for the betterment of society and its mindset over social issues.

Without any doubt, they have contributed the best way possible to change the mindset of people towards the crime that has been going on in society in the name of culture and tradition. The citizens of the country are now well aware of what culture should be taken to the next generation.

Suggestions

Education
Education is considered as the key to all the evil that prevails in the society. A big part of India is dominated by the rural areas where

dowry deaths are more common. Education not only helps in breaking such unlawful customs and practices, it breaks the stereotypes of associating girl child with dowry. Not only that, if a woman is educated, she has the courage to walk out of the torture of her husband and live freely. It is observed that women refuse to report dowry because they do not want to consider themselves as a burden by going back to their parent's house. Legislations will fail if the mind is corrupt.

Gender Sensitization

In order to break the cycle of dowry, it is important to make the genders aware about their role, responsibility and the most important, a sense of equality among all. If the woman is not given due respect, she will always be at low pedestal and will be the means of attaining dowry and fulfilling the demands of a male child only. Gender sanitization should target from the practices like female infanticide, domestic violence and all kinds of crimes against woman.

Strict Laws

The laws need to be amended time and again to fulfill the prevailing needs of society. Lesser number of convictions, lack of quick action, traditional investigation techniques, and outdated laws makes it difficult to curb the problem of dowry. Often dowry is demanded in the name of custom which has no backing, hence, preference should be given solely to law and not to any custom which is against the moral practices of a society.

Women Police

It is worthwhile to empower the women police units to undertake investigations in the dowry related cases, as the women police would be able to effectively understand the sensitivity involved in such cases.

Lack of Awareness

Formation of rules is not enough unless people are made aware of what is right and what is wrong. Social media campaigns, advertisements, and legal aid camps not only make the people aware but they create a fear in the mind of people relating to the consequences of not just taking dowry but also giving dowry. Empowering women plays a very important role. If the woman is not aware of her rights, she fails to raise voices against the torment she faces every day.

Conclusion

"DOWRY IS ILLEGAL BUT SOCIALLY ACCEPTED NORM"

Just like everyone, women also dreams of a perfect life, but what is the definition of a perfect life for a female? For some, it may be a career, however, in India, a majority of females share the dream of a happily married life, with a hope that they will be cherishing the new family and love. However, the evil of dowry is one of the major reasons why the Indian parents regret giving birth to a girl child. They consider the baby girl as a sin, a responsibility, and a shame. This society is made by us and for us, the question still prevails in the nation that why do we need to sell our daughters? Dowry is not just a one-time exchange, if the dowry is taken or given, there is no end to it, with time it becomes the habit of the groom's family. In India, marriage is considered to be a sacred ceremony which is now not less than a business deal, and gifts are no more exchanged as love. It not only prevails in the weaker or uneducated sections, even the rich and educated demand more as per the standard of their livelihood. The enactment of the Dowry Prevention Act in 1961 by the Central Government has even futilely checked its development, to a great astonishment that the state is no better in the 20th century, and we have sunk more in the depth of this evil. The state of this crime in Indian mentality forces us to admit that, it has been there, it is there and it will be. However, this needs to stop, the chain needs to break, laws need to be strict towards the dowry demands, and women police should be empowered to deal with these issues. Giving birth to a girl no longer needs to be considered as shame. A feamle is the only one who is maintaining everything and also giving birth to new generations. Without them, the society itself will end. The saying "son dies of a bad man, daughter dies of a luck man" must be replaced by "living child is of lucky parents".

References

1. S. Ravikant (2000) *Dowry Deaths: Proposing a Standard for Implementation of Domestic Legislation in Accordance with Human Rights Obligations* Volume 6 Issue 2
2. Sen Swagata (2019) *Dowry Killings: Why Does It Happen and How Can We Prevent It? Right of equality*

3. Kishwar Purnima (2005) *Anti Dowry Legislation; Designated to fail*, Manushi, Issue 148

4. Angela K. Carlson-Whitley, *Dowry Death: A Violation of the Right to Life Under Article Six of the International Covenant on Civil and Political Rights,* Volume 17

5. Laursen and Kaur (2013) *Signs of Change: Sex Ratio Imbalance and Shifting Social Practices in Northern India,*

6. Rao and Bloch (2013) *Terror as a Bargaining Instrument: A Case Study of Dowry Violence in Rural India*

7. Gupta, R. (2020) *Dowry Death;Still a threatening reality,* She the people

8. Uddin, N., Hamna, M. A., Talukder, E. ., & Ahmed, R. (2019) Comparative Study on Dowry System. *The International Journal of Social Sciences and Humanities Invention, 6*(11), 5724-5730.

9. Leila Ateffakhr (2017) Dowry System in India; Int J Sci Res Publ 7(3) (ISSN: 2250-3153).

10. Mithun, T. (2018) Dowry System and its Legal Effects In India-A Study; International Journal of Pure and Applied Mathematics Volume 120 No. 5 2018, 1683-1694.

4

Women Welfare and Protection through Women Run Police

Subesha Banerjee

Abstract

Women in India have been guaranteed equality in all spheres by the Constitution. Adding to it, they are granted protective discrimination taking into consideration their plight before independence. Time and again various welfare schemes are made to protect them and empower them for their overall development. Yet, we see crimes against women are rampant. The requirement right now is to enable a complete change in the overall mindset and attitude of the people in order to bring in overall development of a women without any discrimination, thereby, helping them in their empowerment.

Introduction

Gender equality is a basic human right. Every human being is entitled to live a life with dignity and freedom without any fear or favour. In a country like India, protecting and empowering women is indispensable towards development and advancement, thereby reducing gender inequalities, under development, poverty and corruption[1].

As the saying goes 'Mother is the first teacher of a child', therefore, it is important to educate the mother as she leads from the frontline for generations to come. If they are educated, they can contribute more towards the productivity of the whole family as well as the community as a whole.

Sadly, even at this 21st century, discrimination against girl child is rampant. The constitution of India guarantees equal rights to both men and women and stringent laws have been made to stop various

---

[1] Sepúlveda, J. (2003). *The Life and Times of Willie Velasquez: Su Voto es Su Voz*. Arte Público Press.

evil traditional practices. Yet in reality, it takes various forms. Some of the girls are traumatized as a result[2].

Not only discrimination but we also see violence against women. It is committed against women of any age, caste or creed. It is of various kinds – abuse, molestation, rape, infanticides, dowry death, forced prostitution, women trafficking, domestic violence, and abduction.

Crimes Against Women

It is the menfolk who perpetrate nine out of the ten crimes committed against women. This itself proves how these crimes originate as it stems from the deep-rooted patriarchal ideology in the minds of men. From generations, this belief is rooted in the men that the male is physically superior than the female due to which India has now become one of the most vulnerable countries when it comes to numbers and amounts of crime committed against women. Now-a-days, violence against women encompasses physical, sexual, emotional and mental abuse. The violence is mostly carried out by men and it is of great concern[3]. The concern should be immediately addressed.

One evil that happens organically is demand of dowry from the groom's family towards the bride's family. As per age old tradition, the bride's family is supposed to reward the groom with a considerable amount of money and property. In rural India, the bride, usually belonging to a poor household, is unable to meet the groom's high demand for dowry. Even after fulfilling the demands of the groom's family, the bride is subjected to verbal abuse and physical torture. As a result, we see a considerable number of dowry deaths in the rural parts of India. This is one of the reasons why some people kill their young daughters because they know they would not be able to arrange dowry at the time of their daughter's marriage. This leads to the increase in the number of female infanticide (or foeticide) other than discrimination.

---

[2] Beard, M. (1987). *Woman as a force in history: A study in traditions and realities.* Vani Prakashan.

[3] Shrestha, A. P. Domestic Violence against Women in Nepal: Concept, History and Existing Laws.

India has an alarming trend that sees many women die on an everyday basis as a result of harassment over dowry[4]. The woman is either killed or compelled by her in-laws and relatives of the husband to commit suicide[5].

There are so many dowry death cases pending in India. Lots of questions are raised like: are gold and money more valuable than a woman's life? There are many cases that go unreported. Taking and giving dowry has been criminalized by law long time back in 1961. Yet, we see that a large number of families, even in urban areas, openly defy laws and fail to protect women. Strange it is as we get to see educated people living in cities and towns harass women for not bringing enough money or gold from her parents' homes. There are innumerable cases of abuse and death of women for dowry. Thus, one wonders when this plight of women will end.

Patriarchy and Gender Discrimination

Even though dowry system is abolished in India, yet the reason for the prevalence of this custom is because of our patriarchal society which values men over women[6]. The stronghold of the gender inequality in Indian society makes a bride's family feel obliged to meet the dowry demands of the man who has agreed to take care of the daughter[7]. The fact that this dowry system is too deeply rooted in the Indian cultures that it is seen normal and unchangeable. It is considered to be an age-old custom due which many people, even the educated ones, ignore it knowingly. According to Indian culture, a woman's marriage is of paramount importance. Dowry death is basically the result of molding of the Indian traditions and customs. The groom's family take undue advantage of the stronghold of the dowry system which will ultimately bring them wealth. Therefore, it is considered as a duty of the bride to bring dowry along with her. In

---

[4] Scaria, M. (2006). *Woman, an endangered species?*. Anamika Pub & Distributors.

[5] Murthy, P., & Smith, C. L. (2010). *Women's global health and human rights*. Jones & Bartlett Publishers.

[6] Blunt, E. (2010). *The caste system of northern India*. Gyan Publishing House.

[7] Rudd, J. (2001, September). Dowry-murder: An example of violence against women. In *Women's studies international forum* (Vol. 24, No. 5, pp. 513-522). Pergamon.

today's age, it haunts many girls who want to have an empowered and independent life.[8]

The day a daughter is born in the family, either she is considered as a burden or the family starts accumulating wealth aside for daughter's dowry rather than investing in her education[9]. Wonder how long women will have to bear the weight of patriarchal traditions like this. It takes an open passage because no one dares to take legal action against the families.

Now let's discuss about child marriage. Post-Constitution laws and prevalent customs of India have come into conflict with each other over the decades. Child marriage has been declared illegal according to the provisions of the Prohibitions of Child Marriage Act (PCMA), 2006. This law seeks to prevent the solemnization of child marriages. It also includes the prohibition of marriages of children below the age of 18 years for a girl and 21 years for a boy.

As a girl child is considered a burden, the attitude of many families is that it is better to marry off the girl as soon as possible. The reason cited sometimes is that the earlier you marry off the girl child, the lower the cost of dowry. Therefore, she hardly spends time with her parents. In various communities, where the practice is widespread, the conventional belief is held that marrying off a girl child would prevent her from being subjected to male attention or any form of sexual violence, thus, protecting her chastity.

Analysis of Legal Provisions

Initially, the Child Marriage Prohibition Act, 1929 was brought into the statute books as a culmination of sustained pressure by social reform groups and public-spirited individuals who campaigned against the adverse consequences of marriage[10]. This act, however, failed due to various reasons, as the Act itself prohibited complaints after the first year of marriage. Another challenge is convincing the guardians of the children to annul the marriage. Guardians are also

---

[8] www.shethepeople.tv (last visited on 5th November, 2020)

[9] Radhakrishnan, S. (2009). Professional women, good families: Respectable femininity and the cultural politics of a "new" India. *Qualitative Sociology, 32*(2), 195-212.

[10] Harlow, C., & Rawlings, R. (2013). *Pressure through law*. Routledge.

conditioned by societal norms and prejudices surrounding the issue of child marriage. In many scenarios, it is the guardians who push the children into forced marriages at a tender age.

There are inconsistencies with personal laws. As personal laws of certain communities still allow child marriages and the Child Marriage Restraint Act simultaneously tries to prevent them, the conflict leads to significant complications[11].

The Law Commission's report in 2017 titled 'Compulsory Registration of Marriages' and the supreme Court in *Smt. Seema V. Ashwani Kumar* observed that compulsory registration of marriages is each state would be 'a step in the right' direction. The Supreme Court has made registration of marriages compulsory.

Now that states have made registration compulsory, marriage officers and registrars have the duty to intimate about child marriages. Better co-ordination and communication between agencies concerned with the protection of child rights and the statutory authorities, is therefore, the need of the hour.

Women Empowerment through Court Judgments

In the Supreme Court landmark 2017 decision in *Independent Thought V. Union of India*, it was laid down that sexual intercourse by a man with his wife who is less than 18 years of age amounts to rape under the Indian Penal Code, 1860. This judgement not only discourage child marriage as FIRs are registered against many men within child marriages for rape, but also allows child brides to seek relief for annulment.

The groom gets booked under the provisions of both the Indian Penal Code or POSCO for child sexual abuse and the provisions of Juvenile Justice Act, 2000 (in case of minors). This judgement also negatively impacts child brides who voluntarily choose to marry grooms without the permission of their parents/guardians, who, in reaction, file FIRs against the groom to stop the marriage. This independent thought judgement is only the first stop in a long journey to get rid of child marriages in the country. For better implementation

---

[11] Eekelaar, J. (2017). *Family law and personal life.* Oxford University Press.

of the existing laws on child marriage, a proper check on the role of the authorities is essential as they are the first point of contact to prevent such act of marriage.

Child marriage not only affects the basic rights to freedom and life, but also has an impact on the reproductive health of a girl child. The rate of both maternal and infant mortality is high in case of child marriages. This social evil must be rooted out through the legal route, with stricter penal provisions and accountability checks for authorities. Lawmakers and law enforcers must address this issue of vital importance to make sure that children are protected and kept safe[12].

There are a host of other instances of violence which are only increasing. It is ironical that in a land where goddesses are worshipped, the crime are against women is so high. Now-a-days Indian women refuse to be trapped in a bad situation and shed silent tears. Law is a tool for women protection and welfare, which is a must for social change. There are various example to prove that the law have made women eligible for different roles in the world affairs.

Today Hindu women have options to walk out of a bad marriage rather than live unhappily. Several provisions of 'Hindu Marriage Act, 1955' laid down provisions of divorce and empowered the women to say goodbye to their long sufferings. The Act has several provisions relating to registration of marriage, restitution of conjugal rights, judicial separation and various grounds of divorce.

Now women can get a share in the ancestral property due to an amendment in 'Hindu Succession Act, 1956'. There are other laws as well for strengthening the women power, such as Hindu Adaption and Maintenance Act, 1956. As per the 'Muslim Shariyat Act, 1937' a Muslim woman can opt for divorce according to her will and can get maintenance in the form of 'Mehar'[13].

The problem lies in the rural areas where the people are not much educated to be aware of the various laws and legal legislations that take place in the country. Throughout the years, special attention

---

[12]www.thewire.in (last visited on 5th November, 2020)
[13]www. aplustopper.com (last visited on 5th November, 2020)

has been given and steps been taken towards women protection and welfare.

Important Constitutional and Legal Provisions for Women in India

The principle of gender equality is enshrined in the Indian Constitution in its Preamble, Fundamental Rights, Fundamental Duties and Directive Principles. The Constitution not only grants equality to women, but also empowers the State to adopt measures of positive discrimination in favour of women. Within the framework of a democratic polity, our laws, development policies, plans and programmes have aimed at women's advancement in different spheres. India has also ratified various international conventions and human rights instruments committing to secure equal rights of women. Key among them is the ratification of the Convention on Elimination of All Forms of Discrimination against Women (CEDAW) in 1993.

Constitutional Provisions
The Constitution of India not only grants equality to women but also empowers the State to adopt measures of positive discrimination in favour of women for neutralizing the cumulative socio-economical, educational and political disadvantages faced by them. Fundamental rights, among others, ensure equality before the law and equal protection of law; prohibit discrimination against any citizen on grounds of religion, race, caste, sex or place of birth, and guarantee equality of opportunity to all citizens in matters relating to employment. The Articles 14, 15, 15(3), 16, 39(a), 39(b), 39(c) and 42 of the Constitution of India are of specific relevance and importance in this regard.

Constitutional Privileges
- Equality before law for women (Article 14)
- The State not to discriminate against any citizen on grounds only of religion, race, caste, sex, place of birth or any of them (Article 15)
- The State to make any special provision in favour of women and children (Article 15 (3))
- Equality of opportunity for all citizens in matters relating to employment or appointment to any office under the State (Article 16)

- The State to direct its policy towards securing for men and women equally the right to an adequate means of livelihood (Article 39(a)); and equal pay for equal work for both men and women (Article 39(d))
- To promote justice, on a basis of equal opportunity and to provide free legal aid by suitable legislation or scheme or in any other way to ensure that opportunities for securing justice are not denied to any citizen by reason of economic or other disabilities (Article 39 A)
- The State to make provision for securing just and humane conditions of work and for maternity relief (Article 42)
- The State to promote with special care the educational and economic interests of the weaker sections of the people and to protect them from social injustice and all forms of exploitation (Article 46)
- The State to raise the level of nutrition and the standard of living of its people (Article 47)
- To promote harmony and the spirit of common brotherhood amongst all the people of India and to renounce practices derogatory to the dignity of women (Article 51(A) (e))
- Not less than one-third (including the number of seats reserved for women belonging to the Scheduled Castes and the Scheduled Tribes) of the total number of seats to be filled by direct election in every Panchayat to be reserved for women and such seats to be allotted by rotation to different constituencies in a Panchayat (Article 243 D(3))
- Not less than one- third of the total number of offices of Chairpersons in the Panchayats at each level to be reserved for women (Article 243 D (4))
- Not less than one-third (including the number of seats reserved for women belonging to the Scheduled Castes and the Scheduled Tribes) of the total number of seats to be filled by direct election in every Municipality to be reserved for women and such seats to be allotted by rotation to different constituencies in a Municipality (Article 243 T (3))
- Reservation of offices of Chairpersons in Municipalities for the Scheduled Castes, the Scheduled Tribes and women in such manner as the legislature of a State may by law provide (Article 243 T (4))

Legal Provisions

To uphold the Constitutional mandate, the State has enacted various legislative measures intended to ensure equal rights, to counter social discrimination and various forms of violence and atrocities and to provide support services specially to working women. Although women may be victims of any of the crimes such as 'murder', 'robbery', 'cheating', etc., the crimes, which are directed specifically against women, are characterized as 'Crime against Women'. These are broadly classified under two categories.

(1)The crimes identified under the Indian Penal Code (IPC)
(2) The Crimes identified under the Special Laws (SLL)

- Rape (Sec. 376 IPC)
- Kidnapping & abduction for different purposes (Sec. 363-373)
- Homicide for dowry, dowry deaths or their attempts (Sec. 302/304-B IPC)
- Torture, both mental and physical (Sec. 498-A IPC)
- Molestation (Sec. 354 IPC)
- Sexual Harassment (Sec. 509 IPC)
- Importation of girls (upto 21years of age)

Although all laws are not gender specific, the provisions of law affecting women significantly have been reviewed periodically and amendments carried out to keep pace with the emerging requirements. Some acts which have special provisions to safeguard women and their interests are:

- The Employees State Insurance Act, 1948
- The Plantation Labour Act, 1951
- The Family Courts Act, 1954
- The Special Marriage Act, 1954
- The Hindu Marriage Act, 1955
- The Hindu Succession Act, 1956
- With amendment in 2005 Immoral Traffic (Prevention) Act,1956
- The Maternity Benefit Act, 1961 (Amended in 1995)
- Dowry Prohibition Act, 1961
- The Medical Termination of Pregnancy Act, 1971
- The Contract Labour (Regulation and Abolition) Act, 1976
- The Equal Remuneration Act, 1976

- The Prohibition of Child Marriage Act, 2006
- The Criminal Law (Amendment) Act, 1983
- The Factories (Amendment) Act, 1986
- Indecent Representation of Women (Prohibition) Act, 1986
- Commission of Sati (Prevention) Act, 1987
- The Protection of Women from Domestic Violence Act, 2005
- The Plantation Labour Act, 1951

The Present Situation

In spite of many thoughtful Constitutional Provisions and never-ending legislations undertaken by the central government and state agencies, the country has time and again failed as a nation to take care of its women population. Crime against women is still rampant, and there are certain crimes which are present both in the rural as well as in the urban areas[14]. Some of such crimes are women trafficking and forced prostitution, molestation and rape, domestic violence and murder and most importantly discrimination[15].

Trafficking is a trade of humans for purpose of forced prostitution, slavery, labour, etc., and women are often subjected to such evil by their foster father or even by their own parents and loved ones. Molestation is sexual assault or abuse of a person, specially a woman or child. Domestic violence means violent or aggressive behaviour within the home by the husband or the relatives of the husband. Murder means unlawful killing of a human being by another. Steps are being taken to get rid of all such evils and protect the women of India. Various welfare schemes are also undertaken to help them out from various issues in their day-to-day life.

The **Rastriya Mahila Kosh** was set up in 1993 to make credit available for lower income women in India. Various welfare schemes are
i)   **Mother and Child Tracking System:** Launched in 2009, it helps to monitor the healthcare system to ensure that all mothers have access to a range of services, including pregnancy care, medical care during delivery and immunization of children.

---

[14]George, S. (1989). *How the other half dies.* Rowman & Littlefield Publishers.
[15]Fernández-Kelly, M. P. (1983). *For we are sold, I and my people: Women and industry in Mexico's frontier.* Suny Press.

ii) **Pradhan Mantri Matritva Vandana Yojana**: The programme, which began in October 2010, provides money to ensure the good health and nutrition for pregnant and lactating women aged 19 and over for their first two live births.

iii) **Rajiv Gandhi Scheme for Empowerment of Adolescent Girls - Sabla**: Launched in 2012, it offers a variety of services to help young women become self-reliant including education, health and other life skills.

iv) **National Action Plan for Children**: Initiated in 2017, this scheme was launched by Ministry of Women and Child Development.

v) **Digital Laado - Giving Digital Wings to daughters**: This is to empower and strengthen daughters on a digital platform. They just need to register themselves to avail a variety of benefits from this scheme[16].

vi) **Beti Bachao, Beti Padhao**: This is basically a campaign of the government that aims to generate awareness and improve the efficiency of welfare services for girls in India.

Role of Women Police

In a country where women are considered as a goddess by majority of people, it becomes the duty for the authorities to uphold her respect, chastity, integrity and motherhood. For this purpose, women police is employed at various police stations. However, the number of women in police force is extremely low and constitute less than ten percent of India's police force. Yet they play a very crucial and important role when it comes to their role play as women police in a masculine occupation.

In order to maintain peace and tranquility, police are empowered with several powers to prevent and detect crimes and prosecute criminals. Gradually with time, the role and duties of women police has widened and they have ventured into various ranks in order to enforce the law. Their main duty is to be confident and equipped enough so as to deliver support and protection to the victims.

There are many instances where crimes against women go unreported. The victims do not feel comfortable going to a police station

---

[16] www.wikipedia.org (last visited on 6th November 2020)

filled with men police only. In such a case, the victim feels unsafe and ashamed, thus, giving space for the criminals to roam free. The presence of women in the police can help a lot of women who fear social stigma.

Therefore, a lot of women are aimed to be employed in various police stations and the number is increasing along with the police stations. This is also a measure towards equality of sexes. Not only are they being empowered being employed at the police force, but they can also protect victims of violence and can reach out to the most vulnerable victims. Naturally, a woman victim feels more comfortable if there are women around her and is able to open up and divulge all that is required for that case. The main aim is to empower the women folk so that they get the confidence to approach the police without hesitation or fear.

Conclusion

As per various legislations, many criminal cases and especially sexual assault cases are to be recorded and investigated by a woman police officer. A woman cannot be arrested at night, and if arrested during the day, a woman police officer should be present. In addition, the search of women (and juveniles) must be done by the woman police only. In some respects, women are better suited to police work than men. Women police can reach out to the women victims effectively. Therefore, more recruitment and promotion of women police is the need of the moment. A systematic planning must be made to increase in the overall representation of women in policing so that their intervention increases in order to achieve protection and welfare of women. A lot has been achieved, yet a lot needs to be done. More recognition should be given to them and their work.

In every field, overall development of a person is of paramount importance. For women in India, recognition is not even given to the work they do at home. What needs to change is society's mindset and attitude towards women, i.e., a major change of heart. Once total development of a woman is emphasized and exception is achieved properly from all respects, empowerment will follow automatically.

5

The Challenges in Achieving Women Empowerment and the Role of Women Police

Sohini Das

Introduction

The word empowerment ascertains self-empowerment which is a combination of internal-realization or self-realization, power of autonomy, accessing resources, freedom to access opportunities, motivation and power to have control over own life. Empowerment is purely based on some crucial internal factors such as self-esteem, self-control, etc., as well as external factors like liberty to opt for the alternative of own choice, providing motivation for self-reliance, decision making, etc.[1]

We all have the right to pick the substitute suitable for us. For this, we need to possess a strong will power and self-reliance. We must remember that we are human beings with independent will, rational thought and different choices. Empowering someone denotes uplifting the person in each and every aspect of life no matter what obstructions come into the paths of the life cycle. Endearing and approving the will power and autonomy of a person implies the idea of empowerment. In other words, empowering refers to facilitating one's capability and capacity of decision making, choosing the right path in life, enhancing self-judging potentiality and widen up the circle of opportunities.

India is a country of diversity and versatility, and the multiplicity has sprawled in every bit of our country irrespective of caste, class, region, culture, clothing, food habits, norms, tradition,[2] etc., but a common factor that was prevalent all over in ancient India is inequality of power and status in genders[3]. The women belonging to

---

[1] Weissberg, R. (1999). The politics of empowerment. Greenwood Publishing Group.

[2] Keane, J. (2003). Global civil society?. Cambridge University Press.

[3] Sen, A. (2001). The many faces of gender inequality. New republic, 35-39.

higher class were exempted from such inequalities. In history, the evidence of the distinguished women Maitrayee, Gargi and Apala is rife[4]. These venerable ladies notched the mark of education and equality in men and women in Vedic period. The old testaments also witness that the ancient India was devoted to the women and the Indians worshipped the women as DEVI.

In Buddhist and Jainism periods, the stone of gender inequality was planted which was carried forwarded since the later period of Vedic age. During the Mughal period, the misery of women rose to the peak point of discrimination[5]. Purdah, a custom of veiling women, was the first initiative of isolating women from the whole world. The custom of hiding face was engrossed in the whole society[6]. The dream of basic education was elusive for them. Owing to illiteracy, the women in our country in medieval period became entirely dependable on men, and as the only source of bread-earning, the male members of families were prepared to cut down the freedom[7] of the females[8]. All these restrictions and limitations gave birth to some evil malpractices like Sati custom, Child Marriage, Jauhar, etc., which were a great burden for the overall growth and advancement of our country. Ishwar Chandra Vidyasagar, Raja Ram Mohan Roy and Dayananda Saraswati are some eminent personalities of that time who took efforts to eradicate the miseries of life that the women were afflicted with[9]. They explained and deployed the majesty of education for women empowerment. Though they were successful to some extent, yet the women empowerment remained intangible to a large extent.

---

[4] Haddad, Y. Y., & Findly, E. B. (Eds.). (1985). Women, religion, and social change. Suny Press.

[5] Iftikhar, R. (2016). Indian Feminism: Class, Gender & Identity in Medieval Ages. Notion Press.

[6] Chattopadhyaya, K. (1982). Indian Women's Battle for Freedom. Abhinav Publications.

[7] Sinha, J. B. (2014). Psycho-social analysis of the Indian mindset. New Delhi: Springer India.

[8] Forbes, G., & Forbes, G. H. (1999). Women in modern India (Vol. 2). Cambridge university press.

[9] Yousuf, L. (2008). Indian Women: Gender Discrimination and the Governmental Initiatives (Doctoral dissertation, Aligarh Muslim University).

It is a misfortune that women still lagged behind compared to other countries. The earlier mentioned social reformers left no stone unturned to uproot the misconducts impeding the glory of women. Unfortunately, their efforts were not entirely successful. Still, women in our country are not free to choose their life path. In fact, the cases of women trafficking have noticeably increased in many states. The women are considered like marketable products and a lump sum amount is determined for the illegal practice of women trafficking. The concept of worshipping the women as DEVI is no longer subsistent here.

Gender discrimination or rather weakening the women has direct and indirect influences on the economy[10] of a country[11]. A country with gender disparity has imperceptible effects such as increased maternal mortality rate (MMR), child mortality rate (CMR), poverty, population, etc. Moreover, gender discrimination results in high crime rate in a state as well as a country[12]. Female infanticide, women trafficking, domestic violence, etc., are some of the conventional crimes that assert the miseries and distress of women. In search of the causes of such distress of women, the factors come into surface are:

- Scarcity of basic education
- Malnutrition and Poor Health
- Lack of self-esteem and self-reliance
- Superstition
- Lack of Motivation

Necessity of Women Empowerment at a Glance

To Strengthen the Economy of a Country
Gender inequality is very common in developing and underdeveloped countries. The economic status of a country can never be developed without the support of women[13]. If all women of a country

---

[10] Bergmann, B. (2005). The economic emergence of women. Springer.
[11] Dollar, D., & Gatti, R. (1999). Gender inequality, income, and growth: are good times good for women? (Vol. 1). Washington, DC: Development Research Group, The World Bank.
[12] Neumayer, E., & De Soysa, I. (2007). Globalisation, women's economic rights and forced labour. World Economy, 30(10), 1510-1535.
[13] Boserup, E. (2007). Woman's role in economic development. Earthscan.

join their hands with the men in earning their livelihood, then the economy of that country will automatically begin flourishing[14]. The good news is, the participation of women in earning has notably grown in India over few years. Between years 1971 to 1995, the participation of women in labor market had notably increased by 15 percent in Latin America and East Asia which beat the pace of men's participation in labor market[15]. In the course of past fifty to sixty years, life expectancy of women has been increased in developing countries which points out the advancement of women.

To Reduce MMR (Maternal Mortality Rate)

It has been a major worldwide health challenge which is mostly prevalent in developing or under-developed countries where socio-economic status is not up to the mark. Due to complication in pregnancy, a large number of women die every year in India, at the time of pregnancy or child birth[16]. Poor socio-economic condition is one of the active cause of such tragic consequence of women in India. Economically weak people are unable to seek advanced medical aids and proper nutrition for the future mothers that can end up in death[17]. Hence, women empowerment can play a crucial role in cutting down the alarming rate MMR.

To Break the Cycle of Poverty

Women empowerment and poverty have a negative correlation with each other. If one increases, the other will automatically decrease[18]. Poverty leads to crimes like sexual exploitation, women trafficking, etc., that indirectly denote lack of women empowerment. On the other hand, women in developed countries are empowered to choose their life and profession, which marks more income and bal-

---

[14] Rai, S. M. (2013). Gender and the political economy of development: From nationalism to globalization. John Wiley & Sons.

[15] Mason, A. (2001). Population change and economic development in East Asia: Challenges met, opportunities seized. Stanford University Press.

[16] George, S. (1989). How the other half dies. Rowman & Littlefield Publishers.

[17] Bhatt, E. R. (2006). We are poor but so many: The story of self-employed women in India. Oxford University Press on Demand.

[18] Wibbelsman, M. C. (2004). Rimarishpa Kausanchik: Dialogical encounters. Festive ritual practices and the making of the Otavalan moral and mythic community. University of Illinois at Urbana-Champaign.

anced financial condition. This, in turn, makes it possible to eradicate poverty.

To Retrench the Crime Rate

Each and every beat of women empowerment is connected to diminishing crime rate in a country. Gender-based violence in India is
continuing to rise and has already set a benchmark. It suggests empowering women is essential to retrench the crime rate. Domestic
violence, gender determination, sexual harassment, women trafficking, dowry, etc., are a few categories of crime faced by women.

To Enhance the Rate of Literacy

First Prime minister in Independent India (1947-64), Jawaharlal
Nehru, once said, "If you educate a man you educate an individual,
however, if you educate a woman you educate a whole family.
Women empowered means mother India empowered". When the
women will explore their role outside of the kitchen and contribute
financially to their families, the national economy will get a level up.
Therefore, increasing development of women of a country would
result in increasing access to education.

To Increase the Decision Making Capability

For years women are being suppressed by the male dominated societies. It is really unfortunate that even after 74 years of independence, India is still lagged behind in terms of women development
and freedom. A major proportion of India's women are victim of
gender discrimination[19]. They have limited rights to choose their
career path and life partner. Many of them even don't have the right
to put suggestions regarding the family matters. Until and unless the
women have contribution in the society, they would never be able to
take decisions about their own lives.

Challenges in Women Empowerment in modern India

Since independence in 1947, no noticeable drastic change has been
visible in the condition of women in independent India. We need to
remember that no society can develop economically until and unless
the resources are equally accessible to both men and women. A few
factors that interrupt the development as well as empowerment of
women are described here.

---

[19] Schneir, M. (2014). Feminism: The essential historical writings. Vintage.

Poor Economical Background

A large proportion of women in India is housewives and not even interested to engage themselves in office work or business. As a result, our country is incapable to use them as valuable resources to develop our economic condition. According to a survey, only 29% of women in India have been active to earn their bread-butter.

Unwillingness of Political Parties

India is a male-dominant country, and the instance is clearly shown in the political arena too. It is often seen that most of the political parties seek male faces to lead their parties. Since independence, a plethora of male domination has intensely been visible in Indian politics. Moreover, limited number of seat reservation for females in government job sectors is a strong indicator of male dominancy.

Unbreakable Patriarchy

Indian society is ruled by patriarchy where male is considered as the pillar of the family as well as society[20]. In patriarchic society, males are regarded as the guardians of families, and only they have the authority to move forward the families and societies[21]. The cases of honor killing are an evidence of distorted mentality of our society driven by the patriarchal system. Patriarchy significantly interrupts the development of women.

Law and its Implementation

It is quite appraisable that there are a number of laws in India in order to protect the women. Some of the most important Acts for empowering women are as follows:

The Equal Remuneration Act, 1976: This Act crushes the discrimination in remuneration on the ground of gender. As per the Act, the employers have no right to differentiate between male and female

---

[20] Sev'er, A. (2005). Patriarchal pressures on women's freedom, sexuality, reproductive health & women's co-optation into their own subjugation.
[21] Mernissi, F. (1987). Beyond the veil: Male-female dynamics in modern Muslim society (Vol. 423). Indiana University Press.

workers while it comes to paying salaries[22]. The Act boosts the immunity to female workers deprived at work places which indirectly proclaims women empowerment.

The Dowry Prohibition Act, 1961: The Act targets the evil practice of dowry at the time of marriage in the name of ritual. Dowry has been such a malpractice that has taken the lives of many women as they have been unable to fulfill the monetary demands of their husbands and in-laws. The Dowry Prohibition Act, 1961, has come into force on 20th May, 1961 condemning and prohibiting the evil practice of giving and taking dowry. According to this Act, taking or giving dowry is a crime and a person to be accused in this crime is simultaneously punishable and eligible for fines.

The Immoral Traffic (Prevention) Act, 1956, SITA: The abbreviation of Suppression of Immoral Traffic Act, 1956 was modified in 1986 (ITPA) to be loud against the immoral act of trafficking. According to this Act, any person keeping a brothel or being a landlord of such premises or being a tenant of brothel is punishable for 2 to 5 years along with fine up to INR 2000. The Act also punishes a woman above 18 years indulged in prostitution with extended 2 years of imprisonment including a fine up to INR 1000.

Maternity (Amendment) Bill 2017 came into force on Aug 11, 2017. It is an amendment of the Maternity Benefit Act, 1961 that was passed by Parliament in order to regulate the employment of women at work places for a period of 12-26 weeks before and after child-birth. In addition, a woman can avail an amount of INR 3500/- as medical bonus if she is not paid by the employer during her pre-natal and post-natal period. The leave would be fully paid, and as per the Act, violating the provisions of the Act would be punishable.

The Medical termination of Pregnancy Act, 1971 was passed by Parliament of India on 10th Aug, 1971 to provide medical termination of certain pregnancies which is termed as abortion. The MTP Act was implemented in 1972, and a revised version of this Act came into force in 1975. The MTP Act permits the termination of pregnancies in certain cases with the help of medical experts in order to

---

[22] Davidov, G., & Langille, B. (Eds.). (2011). The idea of labour law. Oxford University Press.

avoid any risk of harming the mother. The medical professionals possessing recognized medical qualifications and training in gynecology and obstetrics are permitted to handle or conduct such sensitive cases.

The Commission of Sati (Prevention) Act, 1987, became vocal for effective prevention of the evil practice of Sati, the custom of burning or burying alive of women with the dead body of her husband. Except for Jammu and Kashmir (J&K), the Act became implemented in every part of India for the sake of prohibiting such misconduct of our society. According to Indian Penal Code (IPC), whoever tries to commit Sati would be punishable by the government. Imprisonment for extended one year or fine or both would be applicable for attempting such abominable practice. In addition, any person in abetment to Sati, directly or indirectly, will be imprisoned for life or fine or both.

The Prohibition of Child Marriage Act, 2006, seeks to prevent and prohibit the child marriages in which either the girl or boy is underaged (girls below age of 18 and boys below age of 21). The Act was introduced in 2006 in Indian legislation, however, came into force in November, 2007. The parents of the child or any family member supporting the marriage or negligent in preventing the marriage will be punished up to 2 years with a fine up to INR 100,000 for violation. The girl or boy who has been the victim of marriage has to file the petition in the court to nullify the marriage.

The Pre-Conception & Pre-Natal Diagnostic Techniques (Regulation and Prevention of Misuse) (PCPNDT) Act, 1994, came into operation on Jan, 1994. The Act prohibits the determination of female fetus in pre-natal stage. Not only the diagnosis, but also the advertisement of pre-natal determination and disclosure is considered prohibited under this Act. The person violating the Act comes into conviction under this Act. The act of sex-determination was a prominent indicator of miseries and distress of women in India which has been banned under PCPNDT Act, 1994.

The Sexual Harassment of Women at Work Place (Prevention, Protection and Redressal) Act, 2013, condemns and punishes the offenders who demand sexual proximity, seek physical contacts, and pass sexual remark and other verbal and non-verbal sexual conducts to women at work places. The Act also covers hostile work environment which can be a result of denying or rejecting the sexual proposal made by the higher authorities at work places. Such hostile environment includes, threatening the victim of losing the job, postponing the promotion, compelling the victim to stay at office even after office timing, insulting her without any valid reason, etc. The Act ensures the punishment of the accused after tracing the whole matter. The offenders are required to fill the penalty up to INR 50,000, and continuous sexual harassment can lead to higher penalties and cancellation of business licenses. The Act also ensures punishment for the false complaints.

Indecent Representation of Women (Prevention) Act, 1986, was introduced in order to prohibit and prevent the indecent representation of women in advertisements. It aims to ensure no indecent representation of women in advertisements, publications, writings and illustrations.

Indian legislation has been enacting multiple numbers of Acts in order to stir up the population of our country. However, the proper implementation of these Acts is still out of reach. Most of the times, the patriarchal society plays a crucial role to repress the voice of women. Lack of awareness in women, fear of rejection from the families and society, no other source of livelihood, etc., are some other factors that have played catalytic role in obstructing women empowerment[23]. Thus, the law occasionally fails to enable the women empowerment and diminish the discrimination of gender roles in modern India[24].

Each state police organization is responsible to eliminate the discrimination against women by ensuring the equal rights between both of the genders. The Constitution of India promises providing equality of status and opportunity in Articles 14, 15 and 16.

- **Article 14:** guarantees the equality out of law and does not deny any person to acquire equal protection within the territory of India. The constitution ensures equal rights to human beings irrespective of race, caste, religion, sex or birth place.

---

[23] Verma, A. (2005). The Indian police: A critical evaluation. Daya Books.
[24] Friedmann, W. (1959). Law in a changing society. Univ of California Press.

- **Article 15:** Amended by 93rd amendment in 2005 for providing reservations for SCs, STs and OBCs in private non-aided institutes, this article condemns and prohibits any kind of discrimination based on religion, race, caste, sex and birth place.
- **Article 16:** Ensures equal opportunities in government employment.

After independence, the Indian women expected standard growth and advancement in the societal status. Unfortunately, the minimal recognition in women's societal status is still under the sea in some states of India. The demand of equal rights for men and women has been raised by the women belonging to every part of India. Aiming the overall development, advancement and empowerment of women has been the central goal of government of India. With many activities, the Indian government has been emphasizing on gender equality to uplift the women[25]. In order to meet this particular purpose, the Indian government has arranged the special protection force for prohibiting the crime, offences and discrimination against the women[26]. Despite continuous efforts, the condition and status of Indian women has remained relatively stagnant over few decades.

The percentage of women in law enforcement is relatively less in India as compared to other developed countries such as United States, Australia etc. Women police, the term might give us a jerk, however, the real scenario is that the women constitute less than 13% of total officers in India[27]. Moreover, only a small proportion of women are on higher ranks and authoritative positions. Even there is a limited number of research studies on the topic of women policing, their recruitment, retention, promotion, obstructions and challenges in breaking the stereotype mentality. A few research studies have shown that this career is gaining acceptance slowly in women as this profession is traditionally considered more masculine in nature.

---

[25] Singh, J. P. (2010). Problems of India's changing family and state intervention. The Eastern Anthropologist, 63(1), 17-40.
[26] Misra, L. (Ed.). (1992). Women's Issues: An Indian Perspective. Northern Book Centre.
[27] Sezgin, Y. (2013). Human rights under state-enforced religious family laws in Israel, Egypt and India. Cambridge University Press.

In the era of globalization and women liberalization, the women has started to bloom out in every possible field balancing the personal and professional lives as well. However, manifold challenges and obstructions are still prevalent. The specific challenges ever faced by women police are mentioned in the next section.

Problems and Challenges faced by Women Police

➢ **Challenges faced at work front**

- Owing to late night working hours many women in this profession often face problems due to the society's non-acceptable mentality. For some of them, the families also create a barrier for the same reason as family is a part of the society.
- In this profession, the work load is excessive. It has been found that many of the women personnel quit jobs soon after joining.
- Sexual harassment is reported to be the most challenging cause due to which some officer level women quit their jobs. To be a part of such profession, one has to explore many unknown places to meet new faces. In many cases, the sexual harassment has been the most disgusting nuisance the women police have to face with.
- The profession of police can be very tough for those dreaming of monotonous career options because it needs lots of struggle, going through many hardships and long travel.
- Increasing stress and irritability is something that irrigates the police women. Not only the low graded women police officials but also some higher rank officers have been reported to quit the job due to increasing stress.
- Another crucial point that causes many women not picking this as a career are the health issues. Due to hectic schedule, long working hours, night duty, many with fragile health condition face health obstacles such as eating disorders, sleep deprivation, stress, etc., that frequently lead to multiple health problems.
- The work of a police is always risky and time consuming, but, the remuneration they are paid for the work is not adequate as compared to other professions.
- A survey conducted among the women police shows that lack of basic amenities, such as toilets, uncomfortable duty gear, etc., many times encourages them to quit their jobs.

➢ **Challenges faced at Home**

- Excessive tensions and challenges affect the family life to a great extent. Hindrance to carry out the responsibilities of families and children can sometimes be a very prominent cause behind leaving the jobs for women personnel belonging to the police sector.
- Work schedule, working hours and travel can create a social barrier to women belonging to police sector. Due to lack of social lives, police jobs often lead to stress and tension. Moreover, they frequently become unable to attend or participate in social and religious functions.
- Odd work hours often impede the family lives as well as personal relationships. Due to the heavy work load, the women in police cannot spend time with their families which in turn hampers the personal relationships.

We are fortunate that the non-acceptance in society and various obstructions did not stop our women from opting for a challenging and thorny career path. Thus, many women have elected police service as their profession. In addition, the government of India has come forward taking enough initiatives in promoting women empowerment and equality in every domain of life and profession. There are a number of pathways which promote women empowerment, however, breaking the social hierarchy seems to be very troublesome outside of constitutional and legal reform and socio-economic policy measures. A survey conducted on women witnesses that women feel more comfortable and secured in interacting with a female police officer than a male officer while conveying the violence, discrimination and crimes they have been victimized of. Several studies show that women police are way better in understanding the plight of women and handling violent against women in comparison to male police. Another important point to be noted is that women can speak their heart out to someone who falls in same category in any aspect of life. In other words, women police are representative of women and their empowerment in all sections. Thus, the union government has issued advisories to increase women's representation in policing. In 2009, the union government has adopted 33% seat reservation in police service. In the year 2013, with the revised rule, as per the recommendation of the union government, every police station should have an allotment of at least three women sub-inspectors along with a minimum number of 10 female constables.

Allotment of Women Personnel in Police Force

A rising graph of crime against women in our country has been a subject of concern of central as well as state governments. As per union home ministry statistics, only 3.05% of police force is allotted for women personnel. Uttar Pradesh, the most populous state in India, comprises the police force with only 3.81% women. Tamil Nadu has set an example in this regard, as the Tamil Nadu police contains the highest number of police personnel in India. Andhra Pradesh, Madhya Pradesh and Meghalaya also possess very low percentage of female police. On the other hand, Goa, Himachal Pradesh and Maharashtra are performing well in this regard[28]. The capital Delhi has only 8.64 percent of the police force as women, as per a data collected in 2017. Amid the union territories, Chandigarh holds the better position with respect of women police personnel.

Contribution of Women Police Service (WPS) in Law Enforcement and Women Empowerment

In recent decade, an increasing number of women are joining police force in different cadres to combat with the surrounding environment that gives birth inequality, crimes and discrimination. A strong commitment towards the society has allowed them to plunge into the difficulties and hardships. These women with resilient efforts, indomitable perseverance, and irrepressible bravery have made them susceptible to beat all the orthodox notions continuing since old ages. Indian women in police services are not only working as constables, inspectors or sub-inspectors, but also as higher ranked officers. To explore the world of successful Indian women in this field, we must need to take name of IPS (Indian Police Service) officer **Kiran Bedi**, who has won several awards for her dedication and effort to Indian Police Service. Inspired by her, many other women have tried their fate in police service. She has set an example of women empowerment. Apart from being an IPS officer, she is also a social activist, politician and author at the same time. She has initiated numerous programs against discrimination against women.

---

[28] Chandra Sekhar, A. (2016). Civil Registration System in India-Perspective, Census Centenary Monograph No. 4.

Vimla Mehra was the first women special commissioner of police to introduce a drastic change in women prison as in charge of Delhi's Tihar prison. She induced the foreign language courses in Tihar prison in order to make them self-dependent once they go out of jail. Her other contributions in women empowerment include initiating self-defense training programs for women, introducing women helpline number for women protection, etc. For her never ending contribution and exemplary work, she is considered as a yardstick of women empowerment.

Another ardent example of taking stand against atrocities on women is the women IPS officer **Chhaya Sharma** who investigated the notorious Nirbhaya gang-rape case and was able to bring justice by punishing the culprits. The four convicts in this case were hanged to death in Delhi's Tihar jail in 2020. Despite the difficulties, she cracked one of the most talked about cases and brought justice for Nirbhaya. For her breakthrough success in solving Nirbhaya case, the whole India salutes her.

Meera Borwankar, a woman IPS officer of Maharashtra cadre, is known for her breakthrough contribution to women empowerment. She investigated and cracked the much publicized Jalgaon case, which was a major case of human trafficking, sexual slavery, rape and blackmailing. The scandal came into light in 1993 when few girls filed complained in the police station. Meera Borwankar detangled the whole issue effectively, which involved many prominent personalities.

Another inspiration for thousands of girls was IPS officer **Kanchan Chaudhary Bhattacharya**, the first woman Director General of Police (DGP), who breathed her last in 2019. One of the her most notable achievements was promoting the women and securing more reservations of women in police force. Due to her initiatives, the women home guards were given the responsibility of manning traffic points. She always became voiceful for women empowerment and ensured more training and continuation of women in police service.

Till recently, female in India could not even think of growth and advancement in their status seen today. A few research studies have shown some promising consequences of women empowerment, however, the pace of empowerment is not as rapid as expected. However, a decent number of women are now ready to join police force and many of the existing higher ranked police women have already curved a niche in their respective areas, thus, indicating women empowerment. Hopefully, the number and desire of joining police force would increase in future.

Women Police Station

Vanitha Police Station, located in Kozhikode, a coastal city in Kerala, enjoys the pride and acclaim to be the first all Women Police Station in Asia. It was inaugurated by then prime minister of India Mrs. Indira Gandhi on Oct 27, 1973. Since then, the necessity of all women police stations for eradicating the crimes against women has been prominently realized by the central government of India. A female victim of sexual harassment or rape case can never be that spontaneous in front of a male police. After the first all Indian women police station in Kozhikode, the overall number of all-women police station in India had increased to 479 by 2013.

Matters Looked After by All-Women Police Station

- Investigating and solving of dowry related cases
- Tracing the lost women children and looking after them until their guardians are traced
- Investigating IPC cases related to women
- Providing guard for female prisoners
- Counseling the women involved domestic disputes

Discrimination, Harassment and Domestic Violence Faced by Women Police

Gender discrimination not only attacks the common women, besides, it also victimizes the saviors and protectors of women rights and equality. Despite being in law enforcement, the female cops still suffer from gender discrimination and sexual harassment at their own work place. Many cases of indecent proposals from higher authorities have been reported till date. Shockingly, no legal actions have been generally taken against the offenders. As far as the promotion is concerned, many cases of sexual harassments come in forefront. Disagreeing with the proposal often causes the promotion to be delayed for a long time period. Thus, moving into the higher rank becomes illusive to them despite of their hard work, efforts and significant contributions[29]. Further, most of the time, the male officers are assigned to take up and crack complex cases so that the whole credit could be absorbed only by him.

Discrimination not only arrives from work front, but also comes from their families. Leaving us in shock, a survey made on the basis of women being victim of domestic violence shows that a small fraction of women police have also been enduring violent behavior from their husbands and in-laws. In many cases, police women are married to male officers of the same field and are tortured by their husbands. In addition, they are also not able to complain about this to the police.

These are just some instances based on few survey results, however, more investigations are needed to portray the status of women police in India. For mitigating the internal criminal activities within police services, state as well as well central government need to be aware of these situation and should take appropriate steps. If women in uniform are not safe and are at greater risk of such discrimination, then how can we expect women empowerment within our country?

Status of Women in Different States in India

The southern parts of our country seem to be more progressive and concerned with respect to women empowerment. Karnataka has announced the free access to education for the females from kindergarten to post-graduate level. Such initiatives taken by Karnataka government need to become influencers and motivators in channelizing the spirit and desire of education all over the country.

In India, gender discrimination has been entrenched for years, and the ovation of patriarchy has clogged the mind and thought process. Though India has lagged behind in terms of women empowerment, nevertheless some sections of India have demonstrated extreme advancement in this area. Kerala, God's own country, is the clear indicator of silent revolution. In every aspect of life, in every plat-

---

[29] Mutua, M. (2001). Savages, victims, and saviors: The metaphor of human rights. Harv. Int'l LJ, 42, 201.

form of progression, Kerala women have been one step ahead than women belonging to other parts of India. A survey conducted in 1991 demonstrated that Kerala is the only state in India with a favorable sex ratio of 1040. Kerala became the first state in India in securing 50 percent seats for women in the local and state government. In addition, MMR in Kerala is very low compared to other states. From loan facilities for women in different profession to education for women, Kerala has introduced a new world to women.

On the other hand Bihar, Jharkhand, UP and some regions of MP have lagged behind with respect to women empowerment. Many incidents of brutality towards women, gender discrimination, domestic violence, rape, sexual assault, etc., have been reported. In contrast, states like Mizoram, Sikkim and Manipur are way more secure and safe for women. Goa has been risen to fame for being the safest place in India for women and it is women friendly too. Very less or almost no reports have been lodged till date in Goa for any case of molestation, sexual assaults and rape. However, the capita region has not been so progressive for women so far.

Domestic violence has emerged as a social concern in India, which is rising at an alarming rate. Many women have experienced some sort of domestic violence during their lifespan of which only a small fraction sought help or lodged compliant against their husband or in-laws.

After enforcing the Dowry Prohibition Act for many years in India, our country is still not relieved of this so-called ritual of exploiting the bride and her family economically as well as psychologically. Uttar Pradesh, followed by Bihar and Madhya Pradesh have recorded the highest number of dowry cases in India.

Sex determination and abortion is now prohibited in India and is subject to punishment. Nevertheless, the people following and admiring the patriarchal society are yet to break out from the thought of patriarchy. "Gender doesn't matter" is often recited by many of us, however, in reality, there are so many instances that pressurize us to think about the gender issue. Does it really exist or not. We, the girls, often confront such situations where the males get prioritized.

Conclusion

India, a developing country, where female Gods are worshipped as DEVI, where a number of movies are there to boast the women power, where women represent 29 percent of labor force, however, in reality, they are highly oppressed and marginalised. Domestic violence, sexual harassment, physical assault, rape, gender discrimination, etc., have been the regular incidents of the daily lives of the women.

"To be liberated, women must feel free to be herself, not in rivalry to man, but in context to her own capacity and her personality." - Smt. Indira Gandhi

Referring to the statement made by ex-prime minister Smt. Indira Gandhi, we must seek ways that make our women realize their own capacity and talent and search their own way to bloom out their proficiencies.

Every year, 8th March is celebrated as International Women's Day around the world, an occasion used for shouting out the right of women and manifestation of their contribution in each and every area of life. If we observe thoroughly, we can find cluster of examples of women in higher positions in office jobs and other fields too. However, multiple numbers of surveys evince the fact that even many of those women have also suffered domestic violence, sexual harassment or gender discrimination. Even after implementation of various legal Acts, in favor of women, the crimes against women still persist.

Enforcing the law is only possible by awakening the women, otherwise the government Acts introduced to mitigate the crimes against women will go in vain. Hence, only the law enactment or police services are not adequate. We all, irrespective of male and female, need to fight for women and stand by the side of victims of various crimes. Without a mass movement, no changes in society can be possible.

6

Empowerment of Women through Women Policing

Shivang Rawat

Abstract

The objective of human advancement is strongly in connection with supporting the weaker sections of society. Gender equity is guaranteed by the Constitution of India to all. The economic improvement of women is crucial for the continued development of a country. The modern cycles of advancement have changed the situation of women in India. Thus, women are effectively taking part and giving their assistance in different fields, along with balancing their professional and personal lives. In India, various women have effectively overcome the discriminations and taboos and have excelled in the society. The various examples include Indira Gandhi (the former Prime Minister of India), Pratibha Patil (former President of India) Sushma Swaraj (one of the most powerful women if her time in Indian politics), Kanchan C. Bhattacharyya (first female DGP of Uttaranchal state), Mary Kom (won several gold medals in boxing, thus, taking the Indian sports to new heights).

Introduction

Female police in India are changing the level of viciousness against women. However, according to India Justice Report (IJR), an initiative taken by the Tata Trust, just 7% women in India work in the police department. The main concerns over rising levels of violence against women have pressurized the government to make more stringent laws. Women police stations are distinctive development that have emerged in postcolonial countries of the world in the 20th century to address the viciousness against women. The police associations in India have been commanded to take all measures to deal with the victimization of women and ensure equality between men and women. Similarly, each police association is required to undoubtedly ensure the rights to fairness, non-separation, and uniformity guaranteed by the Constitution of India. The Constitution's Preamble provides all residents fairness of status and opportunity

(Articles 14, 15, and 16). For instance, Article 14 states that everyone is equal in the eyes of law. As per Article 15, State shall not discriminate anyone on grounds of ethnicity, gender, or race. Article 16 talks about equal opportunity in public employment. Further, as per Articles 15(3), the State will make special provisions for women and children. In this respect, Domestic Violence Act, Dowry Prevention Act, Protection of Children From Sexual Offences Act and Child Labour Act are some important provisions enacted by the State. This is acknowledged that women strengthening and progression have been smothered due to auxiliary segregation, and it is the obligation of State to take proactive measures to overcome this imbalance. Broadly, the general improvement of women is a focal objective of the Government of India with a public approach focused on the "progression, advancement and strengthening of women". With these rehashed attestations of the State's pledge to gender equality, women police organizations are bound to ensure uniformity at an institutional level, yet in addition sort out the difficulties faced by women. Women will bring exceptional abilities and interesting points of view to empower the police to react better, especially the most vulnerable will be immensely benefitted. A noticeable women portrayal will be an impetus to break the generalization that policing must be dependent on physical (consequently male), coercive, and solidarity to be effectful. When the very authenticity of this model of policing is continually being tried, filling the positions with women is both an independent objective, and, furthermore, a fundamental driver of democracy based responsive and unbiased policing. In 2013, the Ministry of Home Affairs necessitated that each police headquarters should have three women sub-inspectors and ten women police constables and a help desk area where the women victims can get assistance. In 2015, the government came up with an idea of making Investigative Units for Crimes against Women (IU-CAW) at police headquarters. These units are to be established on a cost-sharing premise between the center and the states, with around 15 officials managing violations against women. Of the 15 staff, at any rate 33% are needed to be women.

Appointment Process in Women Policing

Expansion of the number of women police officers must be accomplished through a systematic and phased system. Meeting the state reservation rate can be set as the principal benchmark. Proactive and exceptional measures pointed toward eliminating boundaries and expanding mindfulness, access and certainty of women are indispensable. All the while, it is the obligation of the police authorities to ensure that women from all social foundations can profit from the chances to join the police. Focus on expanding the number of women in the state police administration is needed at all levels. It is vital to follow unprejudiced, normal and consolidated enrollment systems, including opening all posts similarly to men and women and supplanting terms like "lady constable" or "woman police" in the terminology of posts. It would be worthwhile to embrace 33% reservation for women in the administration as the first benchmark.

Measures Taken to Enroll More Women Police Force

Extraordinary measures are needed to guarantee the quota held for women is filled uniquely by women in direct enrollment. In case the positions earmarked for women stays unfilled in an enrollment year, these should be conveyed forward and uncommon enrollment drives should be held to fill the pending openings. Enlistment drives should be run at many neighborhood levels, not just in local base camp. Nearby media and tertiary instructive foundations should be included to enhance women consciousness and enrollment. Coordinated efforts should be made with schools and universities to hold instructive meetings on policing work and vocation openings in the police for women. The mainstream that policing is only meant for men and not for women should be discarded to clear route for women to be assigned to all policing assignments. Expansion in the number of women police work force should be achieved in the areas of police patrolling, traffic obligations and other obligations including direct collaboration with the overall population, with due consideration of their wellbeing and security. Measures should be taken to guarantee that inside a predefined time frame, women would be positioned across levels including police headquarters, subdivisions, areas, exceptional units and state police, to generate a basic and noticeable mass of women pioneers in key policing posts.

Preemptive Measures Taken for the Victims of Sexual Harassment at Workplace

Each police division is bound to completely abolish sexual exploitation against women in their workplace. For such implementation, solid measures are needed for setting up an open interior grievances system. Moreover, institutional help must be guaranteed for women who decide to record criminal objections of sexual harassment. The police must be the first to conform to laws that ensure rights and set a model.

Vishaka Guidelines

The Vishaka Guidelines pronounced by the Supreme Court of India in case Vishaka vs. State of Rajasthan need to be followed, which include the measures directed by the Supreme Court of India with respect to the police's role in investigating the sexual exploitation against women. An inward approach should be created to strengthen the institutional duty and guide the execution of the Act to plainly characterize acts which establish lewd behavior. The required review systems should be recognized. The scope of internal and local committee of the police department should not be unambiguous. Measures should be in place to secure the complainant/witness(s) and their families.

Internal and Local Committees

Appropriate internal and local committees need to be constituted at the accompanying regulatory units, considering the size of the police administration. It should be guaranteed that the chairperson of each internal committee, and local committee as appropriate, is the senior most lady official of the purview, and there should be no obstruction to her position to direct a request in any event, when the involved official is senior in rank to her. The jurisdiction of each internal committee and local committee should be decided and distributed to all police units. It should be guaranteed that there is no institutional block to the privilege of women police staff to document grumblings of lewd behavior, the successful and autonomous investigations into grumblings, the nature of examination concerning criminal protests of inappropriate behavior, the security of the complainant/witness(s), and the option to advance the suggestions of the internal/local committee.

Dynamic measures should be taken to make the women police staff mindful about the different potential approaches to record objections of lewd behavior at the work environment.

Conclusion

In developing countries, the role of women in police is minimal as compared to the developed nations where women get a chance to work and explore in the law enforcement agencies. In the developing countries, women are neglected and considered to be inferior as compared to their male counterpart. India is trying to give ample opportunities to women in policing. A number of recruitment drives and competency tests are regularly conducted by the police departments for the involvement of women in policing. In patriarchal society, for example in India, most of the people have the perception that women are only capable of bearing a child, taking care of the family, and are not supposed to work anywhere except in their own house. There is an opinion amongst a small group of people that police service is not meant for the oppressed sections of the society. This notion is condemnable because everyone should get equal opportunity in applying for any job. Therefore, the selection should be made based on the skills and qualifications. Overall, recruitment of more women in police will bring some positive change in the society and there will be a balance in the police force if they work with their male counterpart.

7

Cybercrime Against Women in India: Research and Analysis

Sakshi Soni
Prachi Mishra

"Can we secure the world from a bloodless war? I'm talking about cyber security. India must take the lead in cyber security through innovation." - PM Narendra Modi

Abstract

Cybercrime is a term for any criminal behaviour that utilizes computers as its essential methods for commission of a crime. It is an offense that is submitted against individuals or social events of individuals with a criminal manner of thinking to deliberately hurt the reputation of the individual being referred to or cause physical or mental harm directly or by suggestion, using present day media transmission frameworks (for example, data network). In this study, we have discussed about the different aspects of cybercrimes in India. The development of Information Technology Act 2000, ensured that the offences related to cybercrimes are dealt under the Act with some judicial decision. With the nature and characteristics of the cybercrimes This study is mainly focused on the cybercrimes against women in India. This study throws some light on the main reasons which give effects to the growth of cybercrimes against women. The study also discusses about the role of women police in combating cybercrime. Also, the authors have carried out a survey and collected statistical data from the girl students of Banasthali Vidyapith. Lastly, the study is summed up with some remedies and suggestions for combating cybercrime.

Introduction

Under the Hindu mythology, women i.e. *'Mohini'* is a goddess and the only female *avatar* of the Hindu god *Vishnu*. According to the customs of the Indian culture, women are considered as the significant part of the society. The Vedas, which are provided in the Indian culture, considered the females as the mothers, the maker or one who give existence to the other as well as loved and respect them as a "*Devi*" or else "Goddess". Women occupied a vital role in the society. However, in the modern era, women are seen and depicted as objects. They are not treated as equivalent to men in the general public.

The similar situation has also happened in the domain of cybercrime. The offenders think that no one will penalise them and they can easily hide their act. The internet, which is considered as the gift of the technology for humans, is now a days also used with the bad intention or with the criminal mind for committing the offence. In 21st century, cybercrime hinders the security and privacy of women, especially in India, where the legal awareness is much prevalent.

Aim

The study aims to:
➢ Explore the nature of cybercrime against the women in India.
➢ Identify the reasons behind the cybercrime through the survey among the youth.
➢ To recognize superlative plan to avert cybercrime againstwomen and girls.
➢ To assess the awareness about cybercrime among women.

Research Methodology

➢ Law journals
➢ Literature review
➢ Survey

History of Cybercrime

The origin of cybercrime can be traced in the year 1820 in France when Joseph-Marie Jacquard, a textile manufacturer, created a loom with the help of a loop process of weaving the fabrics. The employees of Jacquard, under the fear of loss of their traditional employment, disrupted this process to prevent its use in future. This was the first time a cybercrime was committed.

➤ Evolution of Cybercrime

Year	Event
1870	Technologically skilled persons called "Phreakers" hacked Bell Telephone company and extracted secret information.[1]
1960	The term hacker used positively in the artificial intelligence lab of Massachusetts Institute of technology.
1970	Another cyber-crime i.e. cyber-pornography was evolved. This year is also known for telephone interference by John Draper.
1980	For the first time, US based 414 hackers prepared to break into computers of Los Alamos National Laboratory. Besides this, an investigation revealed that Mc Donald's information was hacked by a hacker.
1990	To encourage internet civil liberties, an international organization Electronic Frontier Foundation (EFF) was established. It defends new technologies which it believes to preserve online civil liberties.

➤ Indian Scenario After Information Technology Act, 2000

During the year 2000, the Central Legislature of India passed the Information Technology Act, 2000, the first legislation dealing specifically with offence of cybercrimes. It deals with offences committed in electronic form with computers and networks. However, the term "cybercrime" is neither defined nor expressed under the Act. With the enactment of the IT Act, various amendments were caried out in active laws, i.e., 'Indian Penal Code, 1860', 'the Indian Evidence Act, 1872', etc.

In 2001, a writ petition was filed in the case of *Jayesh S. Thakkar v. State of Maharashtra*[2], complaining about the pornographic websites on internet. The Bombay High Court ordered to appoint a committee to its recommendations and suggestions to protect people from pornographic and obscene material on internet.

During the phase of 2009 to 2010, the cyber-criminals became more skilled in committing cyber-crimes with the progression of social networking sites.

---

[1] M. Dasgupta, *Cyber Crime in India- A Comparative Study*, 2009, pp.27-28.
[2] (2001) Bom H.C., W.P. No. 1611.

In *Vinod Kaushik & Ors. v. Madhvika Joshi & Ors.*[3], the spouse (wife) was held for unapproved admittance to her significant other's (husband) and father in law's email record to assemble proof in a settlement badgering case.

In the year 2015, Section 66A[4] was challenged on the ground that it is against freedom of speech and expression in the matter of *Shreya Singhal & Ors. v. Union of India*[5]. The Supreme Court struck down this section as it was being abused by the police to arrest individuals for posting basic remarks about social and policy centered issues on social locales.

What is Cybercrime?

In the 21st century, technology has become very advanced and computers play an important role in an individual's life. Now a days, individuals access internet on a daily basis. It connects the people across the globe and allows the information to flow freely. However, it also leads to many incidents of crime. The crime which mainly originates through computers and internet is known as cybercrime. Thus, it can be said that computers and internet act as objects to commit an offence.[6] Through the access of internet, the offender can collect the personal information and data and can use these for abusive or mischievous purposes.

The appropriate definition of cybercrime is not defined under IT Act 2000 or any other statute. However, by the further studies, we can conclude the definition as "cybercrime is a term which is generally used for illegal purposes in which computer can be considered as primary source for commission of crime. It is a kind of offence which is mostly done against an individual or a group of individuals with the criminal intention to harm the reputation of individual or cause mental or physical injury whether directly or indirectly."

In the present time, the young girls mostly become the target of the cyber criminals. The security of women is the main concern under

---

[3] (2010) Cr. Comp 2.
[4] Information Technology Act, 2000.
[5] AIR 2015 SC 1523.
[6] https://www.techopedia.com/definition/2387/cybercrime.

the penal as well as criminal laws. However, in the present time, they are still defenseless under the cybercrime.

Pertinently, during the lockdown in 2020 owing to the pandemic situation related with Covid-19, the National Commission for Women has received 54 cybercrime complaints in April in comparison with 37 complaints received in April 2019.[7]

Nature of Cybercrime

In the prior period, it was easy to define or characterise the crime and its nature, thus, to bring it inside the four walls of definition. However, at the end of the day, from Blackstone to Kenny and from Russell to R.C. Nigam, no accurate or ideal definition of crime is found, and the main reason behind it is that the term crime is not a constant term. It resembles like a mirror which reflects the social principles and popular assessment of society at a given time frame. In any case, endeavour is made by law researchers to characterise it. Sir William Blackstone tried to define the term crime as "an act committed or omitted in violation of public law, forbidding or commanding it."[8] In the present scenario, to deal with the crimes, it is a very useful approach. It aims at the role played by the law in a civilized society. Scientific growth, industrial revolution, enhancement of political foundations, training and intellectual illumination of the human being, release of spiritual grip over community and diminishing ethical standard have distorted the configuration of wrong in contemporary world. The methods for carrying out crimes are currently modest and universal. A computer with an internet is the all-time requirement.

Characteristics of Cybercrime
➢ **Silent in nature**: Cybercrimes are mainly committed under the security of one's place. Due to this, there is no need of any physical appearance before the victim. There are no signs of physical severity or fight at scene of wrongdoing, no cry of agony and so forth, which are otherwise the typical signs of conventional crimes. In a majority of cases, the victim would not even realize

---

[7] Revealed by Indraveni K., Joint Director, Centre for Development of Advanced Computing.
[8] "Blackstone, Commentaries on the laws of England, Vol IV, p. 5."

what has hit them. The blow would be quick, quiet and with an exterminator punch.

➢ **Inclusive in character**: The operational peddle in cybercrime is tremendous, and the lawbreakers regard no national fringes. The criminal can demolish the whole economy of other country by sitting comfortably in a distant nation. The concepts related to jurisdiction have become old and inappropriate, as the entire world could be a crime scene.

➢ **No physical evidence or clues**: In a cybercrime, the place where the crime has been perpetrated does not show any physical proof of the wrongdoing. Normal individual cannot understand it, thus, the experts are required to discover, recover, investigate and conclude the digital evidence.

➢ **Creates high impact**: Generally, these type of crimes create intense damage in the life of victims.

➢ **High potential and easy to carry out**: In the present time, the know-how for carrying out the cybercrime is easily accessible in the public domain.

Forms and Law Enforcement Regarding Cybercrime Against Women

"Cybercrime against women is growing at an alarming rate, and it may pose a major threat to the security of person as a whole."[9] In country like India, the expression "cybercrime against women" is inclusive of sexual offence and sexual cruelty on the networking sites. It includes:

➢ **Cyber stalking**: It is a well known cybercrime in the present era. In this, the individual continuously stalks the victim and leaves unwanted messages. The main reason behind it can be obsession, hate, love, revenge or ego, etc. The vast majority of the cases of cyber stalking relate to women, particularly of the age group 16-35. *Ritu Kohli*[10] case was India's first instance of cyber stalking. Ritu Kohli filed a complaint against a person in the police station, who was trying to defame her and was di-

---

[9] "Cyber-crimes against women in India: Information Technology Act, 2000, ShobhanaJeet/Elixir Criminal 47 (2012) 8891-8895, ISSN: 2229-712X"

[10] http://cyberlaws.net/cyberindia/2CYBER27.html

vulging her personal information. IP addresses was followed by the police and eventually captured the guilty party."[11]

> **Morphing**: When an unauthorised person with fake identity downloads the pictures of victim without her permission and subsequently edits, transfers or reloads them, the process is called called morphing. The next step taken by the perpetrator is to blackmail the victim through the threat of exposing the pictures and degrading the victim in the society. The recent *Air Force Balbharti School Case*[12] is an ongoing case of this type where a school student became a victim of such an act. These act can be penalized under IT Law 2000 and also attract Sections 43 and 66[13] . The criminals can also be punished under Section 509 of IPC.

> **Email spoofing**: It is a word used to portray false email action in which the transmitter address and other part of the email title are changed to seem like the email started from an alternate source. It is mainly done to blackmail the victim through images or to extract personal information. In a recent case, the culprit claimed to be a young lady for cheating and coercing an Abu Dhabi based NRI.

> **Cyber defamation**: It is a kind of cybercrime in which the wrongdoer publishes the defamatory or derogative information about the victim. It can be done against the both men and women, but the victims are mainly women. In the famous case *The State of Tamil Nadu v. Suhas Katti*[14], the 'obscene, defamatory and annoying messages' were posted against a divorced lady. The wrongdoer also created an account on the name of victim.

> **Cyber pornography:** It gives the reference to depiction of sexual material on the net. It can be considered as another threat

---

[11] "Digital Identity and Anonymity", International Federation for Information Processing, 2008.
[12] Abhimanyu Behra, "Cyber Crimes and Law in India," XXXI, IJCC 19 (2010).
[13] Information Technology Act, 2000.
[14] "http://www.naavi.org/cl_editorial_04/suhas_katti_case.htm."

to the women. ***DPS MMS case***[15] is a well-known example. Such acts fall in the ambit of IT Act 2000. Besides the IT Act, the offenders can be punished under various other provisions of IPC like "Section 290, Section 292, Section 292A, Section 293, Section 294 and Section 509."[16]

Grounds for the Expansion of Cybercrimes Against Women

During 2015, less than 260 million people in India were connected to internet. This number has increased to 483 million by the year 2018.[17] The statistical data of 2015 reveals that 29% of internet users were female.[18] The rapid growth of internet and comprehensive dissemination of social media have triggered the rate of cybercrime against women. Illegal access to information and data interference are very common and easily doable in today's advanced era of technology. The main causes for the increasing rate of cybercrime against women are discussed below.

> ➤ **Lack of stringent criminal provisions**: The chief causes of continuous development of cybercrime are the lack of effective cybercrime laws in the country. "According to the Indian Computer Emergency Response Team (CERT-In), 27,482 cases of cybercrime were reported from January to June, 2017."[19] The study of the said report shows that a cybercrime has been committed every 10 minutes during the period from January to June, 2017.[20] Despite such tremendous growth, the rate of detection and conviction is awfully low. For instance, out of 10,419 cybercrimes were filed in Maharashtra during the period from 2012 to July, 2017, only 34 convictions were made.[21]

---

[15] http://en.wikipedia.org/wiki/DPSMMS Scandal.

[16] Indian Penal Code, 1860.

[17] https://www.statista.com/statistics/255146/number-of-internet-users-in-india/ (Accessed: 09-Sept-2020)

[18] https://www.statista.com/statistics/750999/india-share-of-internet-users-by-gender/ (Accessed: 09-Sept-2020)

[19] K. Chethan, "One cybercrime in India every 10minutes - Times of India," The Times of India, 22-Jul-2017.

[20] Supra note 1.

[21] J. S. Naidu, "10,000 cybercrime cases, only 34convictions in Maharashtra between 2012 and2017," http://www.hindustantimes.com/, 21-Aug-2017.

The reason behind such low conviction rate is the lack of stringent criminal laws provisions. The Information Technology Act, 2008, which is mainly enacted to promote e-commerce, focuses on commercial and financial crimes. On the other hand, the cybercrimes against women are not given much importance and are nowhere specifically dealt with in the Act. These crimes are generally dealt under "Section 66 (hacking), Section 67 (publishing or transmitting obscene material in electronic form), Section 72 (breach of confidentiality), etc."[22]

> **Lack of high-tech resources**: An investigation of cybercrimes requires high-tech resources and procedural implementation. A lack of these resources makes the detection of cybercrimes and collection of digital evidences more difficult. "There are no standard documented procedures for searching, seizing of digital evidence and standard operating procedures for forensic examination of digital evidence."[23] Thus, India needs to upgrade cyber security cells to combat cybercrimes and impart technological training and specialized skills to its officials to fight against cybercrimes against women.

> **Lack of co-operation between countries**: Beside the high-tech resources and standard procedural implementation, international co-operation among nations is needed. It is obvious that cybercrimes have no international boundaries. It may be possible that the offender sitting in one country targets the victim in another country. Thus, it becomes difficult to detect the offender without the legal assistance and co-operation of other countries. The lack of mutual co-operation and assistance leads to the low rate of conviction and consequently gives rise to the rate of cybercrimes.

> **Sociological reasons**: The analysis shows that very few numbers of cybercrimes against women are reported to the police.

---

[22] Information Technology Act, 2000.
[23] V. Nanjappa, "Conviction rate in cyber crime is 0.5per cent- Here are the reasons,"www.oneindia.com, 02-Jan-2015. [Online]. Available:http://www.oneindia.com/feature/conviction-rate-cyber-crime-is-0-5-per-cent-here-are-the-reasons-1609728.html. [Accessed: 04-Mar-2020].

Thus, the lack of strong laws or high-tech resources are not the only factors behind the growth of cybercrimes. The societal stigma of defamation of victim and her family is heavy on the victim's mind in such cases. The convention of blaming a woman for every act committed against her is also very common. This gives rise to the reluctance of women to even report the cases.

Role of Women Police in Combating Cybercrime

Due to the exponential growth in cybercrime, it becomes important for police to handle these types of cases very seriously. In these type of cases, women police plays an important role and becomes role model for the victims. In the department of police, recruitment of women police also encourages the gender equality and inspires many women and girls to be aware of their own rights. In most of the cases of cybercrimes, the victims are not much comfortable to openly describe the things to the male police officer. The victim can explain the whole incident to female police officer more at ease.

According to United Nations, equality, peace, justice and strong institutions are the vital principle. For achieving these principles, it is important to provide equal opportunity by the agencies to become gender neutral, and ensure justice to women and girls. In country like India, the ratio of recruitment of women police is very less. A low percentage of women makes their job challenging at all ranks. As per the study, it shows that women are 27% times more likely to be abused online than man.[24]

Thus, it becomes very important to recruit more women police officers in the police department for the promotion of 'gender essentialism' and 'feminising of policing'. At present, it is necessary to promote, secure and stimulate the work environment to provide more carrier opportunities for women.

---

[24]   "https://m.economictimes.com/news/defence/women-police-personnel-constitute-a-meagre-8-98-of-police-force-across-india-bprd/articleshow/73736033.cms"

➤ **Recommendations Regarding Women Policing**

- In the police department, it is necessary to develop new strategies to recruit and provide adequate training to more women officers.
- Cybercrime against women should be dealt with utmost priority.
- United Nation Gender Toolkit should be used as a training material.
- In every police station, there must be separate cyber unit for women and girls.
- Regularly review and evaluate the progress of women police officers in their work.
- Updated record of the complaints of cybercrime against women should be maintained.

Survey Results and Analysis

A survey was conducted with a sample size of 500 female students of Banasthali University to analyse the awareness about cybercrime among women. While asking students that how many times they have been the victim of cybercrime, the responses were like this: 6% responded that they have been the victim many times, 9% of them were victim for at least 5-20 times, 31% responded that they have never been a victim, while 54% of them were victim for at least 2-5 times (refer to Figure 1 given below).

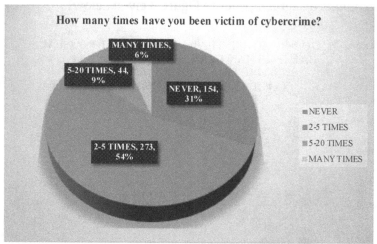

Figure 1

The next question was related to sufficiency of existing laws against cybercrime. Although most forms of cyber-crimes come under the ambit of Information Technology Act, 2000, however, but it is important to know whether the existing laws are sufficient to combat cybercrimes against women. Surprisingly 56% of them responded that there should be enactment of more effective laws, 24% stated that existing laws are partially sufficient. On the other hand, only 20% said that they are sufficient (refer to Figure 2 given below).

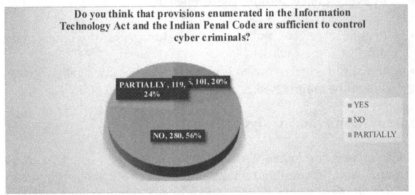

Figure 2

Cybercrimes are committed beyond international boundaries. When asked whether it would be beneficial that an international law rather than a national law should be enacted to fight against cybercrime, majority of the number of students agreed to it and only a few students disagreed (refer to Figure 3 given below).

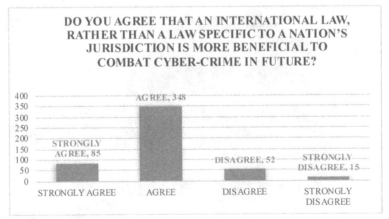

Figure 3

The last question was about criminalization of usage of internet with the object of storage, retrieving and broadcasting sexual content. The number of students who strongly disagreed to is just 28, 57 students simply disagreed. On the other hand, 104 agreed and 311 students strongly agreed to it (refer to Figure 4 given below).

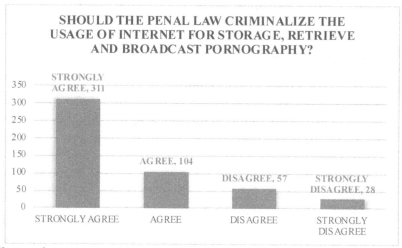

Figure 4

Remedies Available

- "Cyber Crime Prevention against Women and Children Scheme"[25] has been framed by the Ministry of Home Affairs to have an operational instrument to combat cybercrimes against women in India. The scheme includes five components:
    - o Online Cyber Reporting Unit
    - o Forensic Unit
    - o Capacity Building Unit
    - o Research and Development Unit
    - o Awareness Creation Unit
- Police station and cells are established in every state for investigation related to cybercrime.

---

[25] "https://mha.gov.in/division_of_mha/cyber-and-information-security-cis-division/Details-about-CCPWA-CybercrimePrevention-against-women -and-Children-scheme"

- The Ministry of Home Affairs established a portal namely www.cybercrime.gov.in for cybercrime complaints.
- To prevent, detect and mitigate cyber-attack, government has circulated computer security policy and guidelines to all ministries/departments.
- In many north-eastern states and in some cities like Mumbai, Pune, etc., cyber forensic labs has been established by Ministry of Electronic and Information Technology to train state police and judiciary for dealing with cybercrime.

Suggestions to Combat Cybercrime

➢ A collective implementation of measures and initiatives by government and legislative bodies would be effective in combating cybercrimes.

➢ As *"prevention is better than cure"*, to prevent cyber stalking, one should be careful while disclosing personal information and sending personal pictures to strangers.

➢ Awareness and education relating to cybercrimes is essential to avoid such crimes.

➢ Firewalls function as defense in case of online trespass, therefore, these should be enabled.

➢ Society must encourage women to complain about the cybercrimes.

➢ The information technology departments should upgrade their resources to promptly detect cyber criminals.

➢ As cybercrime is a global issue, countries need to collaborate with each other and enact laws against cybercrimes at international level.

Conclusion

The central issue of cybercrime lies in the usual methodology and the diligence of the cybercriminal. The police, legal executive and the analytical offices need to work side by side by employing the most recent advancements with the goal to rapidly recognise the cybercrimes. It is the activity of the legitimate framework and administrative offices to guarantee that the advancements do not become devices of misuse and provocation, To counter cybercrime against women, not just strict corrective changes are required, an adjustment in the training framework is also additionally needed.

References

("Cyber crimes against women on the rise", 2020). The Hindu News. Retrieved   from https://www.thehindu.com/news/national/andhra-pradesh/cyber-crimes-against-women-on-the-rise

Halder & Karuppannan (2016). *Cyber Crimes Against Women in India.*   Retrieved   from https://www.researchgate.net/publication/310774217_Cyber_Crimes_against_Women_in_India

Jain, M. (2017). *Victimization of Women Beneath Cyberspace in Indian   Upbringing.*   Retrieved   from http://docs.manupatra.in/newsline/articles/Upload/786274E9-B397-4610-8912-28D6D03230F9.monika_jain_pdf_1-1111.pdf

Kabir, N. (2018). *Cyber Crime a New Form of Violence Against Women: From the Case Study of Bangladesh.* Retrieved from https://papers.ssrn.com/sol3/papers.cfm?abstract_id=3153467

Misra, R. (2013). *Cyber Crime Against Women.* Retrieved from https://papers.ssrn.com/sol3/papers.cfm?abstract_id=2486125

Pawar & Sakure (2019). Cyberspace and Women: A Research. *International Journal of Engineering and Advanced Technology, 8(6S3).* Retrieved   from   https://www.ijeat.org/wp-content/uploads/papers/v8i6S3/F13130986S319.pdf

8

Women Police Station: Way Forward to Legal Empowerment

Sadaf Moosa

"Real change, enduring change, happens one step at a time." - **Ruth Bader Ginsburg**

Abstract

Gender inequality is the root cause of increasing number of crimes against women. The gender based violence across the globe affects 1 in 3 women and mostly goes unreported. Traditionally, reporting of gender violence is considered social taboo for women. It becomes more difficult for the victim to communicate with the police in the non-conducive atmosphere in the police station. To reduce the gap of inequality in the society, it is pertinent to legally empower women by spreading awareness about their rights and use of legal system. Legal empowerment is the utilization of law, legal procedure and legal aid to safeguard the rights. This article focuses on importance of establishing independent platform to provide easier access to justice through all women police station. This kind of setup ensures a comfortable arena for women to voice their concerns. It is asserted that the All Women Police Station is a little step leading to the legal empowerment of women. The statistics are showing that the women victims reporting offences committed against them has sharply increased in India. The study concludes with few suggestions to make the women police station as an instrument to empower women, accessibility of justice to the victims and prevent gender violence.

Introduction

Women police station is a step towards bringing about change for the empowerment of the women. It will give strength to the women police and courage to the female victims. It is believed that the various global challenges in the changing world can be addressed by empowering women. At current scenario when the violence against the women has been increasing day by day, the establishment and accreditation of women police station is the need of the moment.

The statistics shows that the registration of cases of violence committed against women has increased by "*7.3% i.e. from 3.78 lakh cases in 2018 to 4.05 lakh cases in 2019*". Most of the registrations of the instances in India were "*registered under 'cruelty by husband or his relatives' (30.9%), followed by 'assault on women with intent to outrage her modesty' (21.8%), 'kidnapping & abduction of women' (17.9%) and 'rape' (7.9%). The crime rate registered per lakh women population is 62.4 in 2019 in comparison to 58.8 in 2018*".[1] According to figures of the National Commission for Women in India, in the month of April 2019, it has received 37 cybercrime online complaints while in contrast in the same month in 2020, 54 computer related crime against women has been reported online. The month of March 25 up to April 25, 2020 witnessed the reporting of 412 cybercrimes against women out of which 396 were grievous in nature. This situation calls for the gender sensitization and access to the justice. The All Women Police Station is an effort in the path of legal empowerment and building confidence and trust in women victims. The emancipation of women because of women police station is twofold. Firstly, the women will get due representation in the traditionally male dominated job and, secondly, the women can avail justice by duly reporting the crime, thus, deterring the future crime.

Women Empowerment

The Co-Chair of Gates Foundation and a philanthropist, Melinda Gates opined "*A woman with a voice is, by definition, a strong woman*". When a woman can raise voice against inequality and injustice against her at that moment, she becomes impregnable. Women empowerment is the autonomy to independently decide and make choices. It is an ability to take stance for the right and fight for it, an

---

[1] Jain Bharti, 2020, NCRB Crime Data 2019: Cases registered up 1.6%; crimes against women rise 7.3%; cybercrimes jump 63.5%, https://timesofindia.indiatimes.com/india/ncrb-crime-data-2019-cases-registered-up-1-6-crimes-against-women-rise-7-3-cyber-crimes-jump-63-5/articleshow/78394087.cms

ability to take decisions, an ability to assert or deny, an ability to ask for government amenities, an ability to participate significantly in the society, an ability to check concerns which influence her, an ability to become independent and pursue goals, and to have self-power and self-strength to live a dignified life[2]. The Beijing Declaration at the Fourth World Conference on Women (1995) asserted , *"Women's empowerment and their full participation on the basis of equality in all spheres of society, including participation in the decision-making process and access to power, are fundamental for the achievement of equality, development and peace".* The diverse dimensions of empowerment are as follows:

- Economic empowerment: Women get space to become financially independent.
- Social empowerment: This gives her freedom to live with dignity, educate with confidence and work without fear.
- Political empowerment: Access to voice her opinion and choose the right political leadership who can understand and alleviate her concerns.
- Legal empowerment: Legal system which is enacted to protect her against undue power forced upon her.

Defining Legal Empowerment

Legal empowerment is the application of law, legal process and legal aid to strengthen the rights and interests of the disadvantaged populations like people from weaker society, women, children, etc. The term legal empowerment was introduced for the first time in Asia Foundation report for the Asian Development Bank (ADB) in 2001. It gained popularity by a 2008 report of the Commission on Legal Empowerment of the Poor (CLEP). *"Legal empowerment is empowerment brought about through the use of legal processes".*[3] The foremost aim of legal empowerment is to *"increase access to justice by legal services, legal capacity development, legal and human*

---

[2] Lyda Nyesigomwe , 2012 Empowerment , United Nations Social Development Network
[3] Cotula L (2007) Legal Empowerment for Local Resource Control: Securing Local Resource Rights Within Foreign Investment Projects in Africa 18.

rights awareness and related development activities".[4]   The 2001 report by the San Francisco-based Asia Foundation defines legal empowerment as *"the use of law to increase the control that disadvantaged populations exercise over their lives."*[5]

The establishment of All Women Police Station is one of the stepping stones to make women legally empowered. Women feel at ease to approach police station and report crime committed within four walls of their house or in public. In India, women especially from rural and remote areas still feel shame to complain about sexual offence in front of policemen and fear to be judged as woman of bad repute. With the All Women Police Station, women can exercise their right to live in an equitable society with human dignity by exercising their legal rights.

All Women Police Station: An Innovative Notion

The women police station is a very innovative concept that has gained momentum across the globe. The police station is managed by all women police and focuses primarily on the various crimes committed against women viz. psychological violence, domestic violence, sexual violence and other gender based violence. All Women Police Station also provides financial, medical and mental support to the victims.

The first women police station was established in 1973 in Kerala, India. Thereafter, in 1985, women police stations were set up in Sao Paulo, Brazil.[6] Totally women based police stations are now spread across *"India, Pakistan, Kosovo, Ghana, Liberia, Nicaragua, Peru, Sierra Leone, South Africa, Uganda and Uruguay"*. Several reports from different countries have pointed out that the women have now more trust in police, which has resulted in an outstanding increase in reporting crime as well as high conviction rate. Women policing has

---

[4] UNDP Indonesia (2007) . Project Facts: Legal Empowerment and Assistance for the Disadvantaged.
[5] Golub S And Mcquay K (2010) Legal Empowerment Working Papers, What is Legal Empowerment An Introduction, International Development Law Organization , pg 1-3
[6]   Latin   American   Perspectives,   Womens   Police   Stations, https://en.wikipedia.org/wiki/Women%27s_police_station

had a positive impact in the present scenario as women police can be less judgmental and more female-friendly.

The establishment of the women police station is result of the fact that the relief available from the police station was generally inadequate or sometimes discriminatory. It has been reported that, in Brazil, the number of case of violence against women has seen a steep fall. There has been a 50% reduction in homicide cases of women between the age of 19 to 24. The women officers wear uniforms and carry weapons and enjoy same powers and training, as the general police. However, they operate differently from the traditional police model. Women police officers are deeply embedded in their communities. They are highly visible and welcoming during festivals and protests. Women police stations provide childcare, legal support, social services and psychological support to provide access to justice and mental health to the women and children in one place.

In India as well, the adoption of women police stations led to significant increase in the crime reporting with a 22% rise. Therefore, it led to the rise in arrests of persons accused of committing crime, thus, providing enhanced protection to women.

The effect of women police station is directly related to the process by which it handles the victim and recording of the complaints. The victim does not have to think twice before approaching the women police station. It also gives much better understanding to the police officer, of the grievances of the victim, thus, enabling her to initiate appropriate action against the accused. A female friendly environment gives the victim comfort to open up about her issues without hesitation and request for suitable support from women police officers. The officers are trained in handling and investigating such cases, ensuring speedy justice.

Emergence of All Women Police Station in India

Women police station is a supplementary effort to empower women police force as well as women folks. In the backdrop of the 2012 Nirbhaya case and subsequent nationwide outrage, the government decided to establish all women police station across India. The All Women Police stations were set with the female officers, complete with beat officers on bikes and weapons. This ensures confidence in women so that they can report their grievance or violence committed against them freely. The first All Women Police Station was introduced by Jacob Punnoose, Ex-DGP, Kerala and was set up in Kozhikode in the state of Kerala in 1973. It was inaugurated by then Prime Minister, Indira Gandhi. However, it was later shut down on the ground that it segregates women from rest of the community which was against the interest of the women. Thereafter, in Arunachal Pradesh, the All Women Police Station was established to deal with crimes against women. West Bengal became the next state in India to have such police stations, followed by Andhra Pradesh. The total number of such police stations across India had increased to 479 till 2013.

In India, women police officers are present in regular police stations too, then why there is a need to set up separate All Women Police Station in India? There are several reasons from the perspective of the female police officers as well as female victims of gender violence. The women police officer alleged that they face gender biasness as policing is traditionally considered as a job for males only. The concept of patriarchy is deep rooted in the policing system and, therefore, there is always a question on the capability of the women police in this field. *"The female police personnel were allotted in-house tasks that did not require them to leave the station. They maintain registers, file FIRs, deal with the public and do other tasks while their male counterparts conduct investigations, patrol, and provide VIP security."*[7] Policing has to be fair, free and sensitive to everybody regardless of gender. Sexual harassment at workplace has been reported by the women police. The worst part is *"there was no sexual harassment committee at their workplace, despite such a committee being mandated by the Sexual Harassment of Women at the Workplace Act of 2013"*. The police stations have no separate toilets and changing rooms for female police personnel. Further, there is no maternity and child care facilities for women police personnel at their station.

There is always a shortage of women police officers. In 2009, it was laid down by the government that there should be 33% women's

---

[7] CHRI Report 2018, Model Policy for Women in Police in India, Commonwealth , Human Rights Initiative.

representation in the police.[8] However, till now, the target has not been achieved in several states.

The India Justice Report by Tata Trust was drafted in corroboration with *"Centre for Social Justice, Common Cause, Commonwealth Human Rights Initiative, DAKSH, Tata Institute of Social Sciences - Prayas and Vidhi Centre for Legal Policy"*. The report was published on November 7, 2019 and reported that the representation of women is only 7% of 2.4 million police personnel, prison staff constitute 10% of the women police and approx. 26.5% of judges in high courts and subordinate courts are female. Further, the report disclosed that women police at officer level accounts for only 6 percent of all police personnel. The report stated that *"Even if states commit to increasing women's representation at a modest additional 1 percent per annum, it will take decades to reach even to the aspirational 33 percent."* The report also highlighted that only 6.4% of total police personnel are trained in service during the last five years. This shows that about 90% of police are handling the masses without training on contemporary issues and challenges.

All Women Police Station: A Beacon of Hope

The Thomson Reuters Foundation in its survey pointed out that India is the most vulnerable country across the world for women.[9] The opening of All Women Police Stations has increased reporting of crime by a significant 22% in cases like rape, sexual violence and molestation. The women feel more safe, confident and comfortable in approaching such police stations. The victims do not feel shy to explain the crime committed against them. A report by the United Nations Women (2011-12) named as "Progress of the World's Women: In Pursuit of Justice" stated that *"Data from 39 countries shows that the presence of women police officers correlates positively with reporting of sexual assault, which confirms that recruiting wom-*

---

[8] Government of India, Ministry of Home Affairs, Advisory (2009), F.No.15011/48/2009-SC/ST-W:
https://mha.gov.in/sites/default/files/AdCrime-Agnst-Women170909_3.pdf.

[9] Goldsmith Belinda, Beresford Meka, India most dangerous country for women with sexual violence rife - global poll, Thomson Reuters Foundation, https://in.reuters.com/article/women-dangerous-poll/india-most-dangerous-country-for-women-with-sexual-violence-rife-global-poll-idINKBN1JM076

en is an important component of a gender-responsive justice system." The report pointed out that women find it difficult and unconfortable to approach male police officers. It also noted that *"both male and female victims of sexual violence expressed a preference for reporting to women police."*

A survey conducted in 2015-2016 by the National Family Health, India shed light on the fact that out of the total sexual assault cases taking place in India, 99% are not recorded. It was further observed that *"the rise in the number of policewomen resulted in the decline in rates of domestic abuse and intimate partner crime."* The women police force deals with vivid cases like dowry cases, domestic violence, rape cases, caste based issues, eve teasing, cybercrimes targeting women, etc. The women police also maintain public order and tranquility, as the law requires that only the woman police officers are allowed to physically contact women. Woman police also act as mediators and settle the disputes. They also manage counseling in matrimonial disputes and safeguard families from grievous consequences. They encourage love, respect and bonding among the spouses.

The women police use less physical force than the male counterparts. The Status of Policing 2019 reported that the women police personnel are less likely to use excessive force as compared to the male police officers.

Women have more pro social traits than men. The All Women Police Station can be a ray of hope for many women across the globe. There is a need to build the women police station more women friendly and conducive for the victims.

Suggestions

• It is need of the hour to increase the appointment of women police in police departments. The focal point should be to meet the 33% reservation for women in all categories as early as possible with maximum time limit of 2030[10] and thereafter

---

[10] In fulfillment of India's obligations under the Sustainable Development Goals. United Nations Sustainable Development Goals:, https://www.un.org/sustainabledevelopment/

achieve the target of proportionate representation of men and women at all levels. It is also important to note that the women from all structures of the society should be given equal opportunities to compete to join the police.

- Shy and shame cause distress among women in rural areas. There is a need to set up more All Women Police Stations so that the female victims can get access to women police stations even in remote villages.

- As the gender violence is rising these days, it is necessary to constitute more women police stations. Promotion should be fair, transparent and non-discriminatory.

- Women police personnel should be given proper training to raise their confidence and handle stressful situations. Special training should be imparted to the women police force for the investigation of gender based violence as well as criminal offences committed against children. They should also be trained in information technology and computers to deal with cyber-crime cases. There should be special educators and clinical psychologists to handle the cases of persons with long-term special needs.

- Male police officers should be more gender sensitized through induction training as well as in service training. This will help in building a safe and secure platform for the female victim to go to police stations and report the crime.

- The All Women Police Stations should have all the basic facilities for the female police officials. India has predominantly patriarchal society and women are expected to do all household work as well as to take care of the children, which needs a change. Infrastructure of the All Women Police Station should be women friendly with proper toilets, changing rooms as well as maternity and especially safe and secure child care facilities or crèche as required under the Maternity Benefits (Amendment) Act, 2017 so that a supportive and comfortable work environment can be ensured to the women police. This is the focal point to motivate and keep women in policing and encouraging much more new recruits to join the police force.

- In every police department, there should be committee to report complains in accordance to the Sexual Harassment of Women at Workplace (Prevention, Prohibition and Redressal) Act, 2013.

- It is important to promote and spread awareness about All Women Police Stations. The more women are aware of their rights and its enforcement, the more they will be legally empowered.

Conclusion

The justice system stands on the four pillars viz. law enforcement agencies, penal institutions, independent judiciary and legal assistance. The police are the protectors and enforcer of citizens' rights. The police need to be neutral, impartial and upholder of the rule of law. Inclusion of women in policing supports the other women to access justice. The India's first Prime Minister, Jawaharlal Nehru observed *"You can tell the condition of a nation by looking at the status of its women"*. Women play a major role in building a nation. Women empowerment entrusts more power to take decisions and control the process affecting the life of the women. The initiative taken by the government to establish All Women Police Stations is commendable and a giant step towards the women empowerment. Though there is always an argument that it will lead to the segregation of women and act against the larger interest of the females. At the same time, the women police stations across the globe are receiving a positive response. Hence, it is a meaningful step to the journey of empowerment. An empowered woman can lead to the overall development of a country.

"For we women are not only the deities of the household fire, but the flame of the soul itself." – **Rabindranath Tagore**

9

A Socio-Policy Analysis on the Role of the Welfare and its Contribution in Empowerment of Women through Permanent Commission of Female Officers in the Indian Armed Forces

Purnima Sharma
Shreem Bajpai

Abstract

India, like every other nation, is fighting with the issue of gender inequality. Various steps have been undertaken by the government bodies in the contemporary India in order to empower women and grant them equal opportunities and means to break the traditional and cultural expectations and be at par with men. The decision of the apex court granting permanent commission of women in the Indian Army goes a long way to empower women. The authors through this paper peruse the changes and challenges brought in by the apex court's decision and its role in women empowerment. The paper through a sociological and constitutional analysis of the decision attempts to study its long term effect on gender sensitization in the country. The paper focuses on the role of the Indian Judiciary in strengthening and endorsing participation of women in the Indian military. Lastly, the paper by taking into account the social and political dilemmas of inducting women in armed forces, reads into the limitations and shortcomings and attempts to provide a policy solution for the same.

Introduction

The differential treatment between the two renowned genders has been a pressing issue for as long as one can remember. This differential treatment is often substantiated due to the biological difference between the two genders. In almost every sector, be it economic, political, and administrative, etc., participation of women has been minimal. Increasing this minimal participation by providing equal opportunities and means to the female population of a nation is characterized as '*women empowerment*'. The recent decision of the Supreme Court in granting permanent commission to women in Indian Armed forces is one such ideal example.

Military requires a greater standard of discipline and punctuality and is much more rigid in its operations than any other institution. Composition of women in Indian army, air force and navy combined as per 2018 has been 3,653 women compared to 62,507 men[1]. In order to amend this situation, various initiatives have been under-taken by the government but a proper implementation of the same lacks. There are innumerable authoritative women who had the honor of serving the nation in various forms irrespective of certain (gender) biases and limitations. Some of these brave hearts are Punita Arora, who is presently serving as the Lieutenant General of Indian Armed Forces along with the rank of Vice Admiral of Indian Navy; Lt Col Mitali Madhumita, who was India's first female officer to accept the Sena Medal for gallantry, a decoration given to War heroes for exemplary courage during operations in Jammu & Kash-mir and the northeast; and Priya Jhingan, who was the first lady to be employed in the Indian Army.

The decision of the apex court in granting women permanent com-mission is a definite step towards women empowerment. Through this paper the authors try to highlight the present condition of women in the armed forces and the changes brought by the judg-ment in the armed forces as well the social structure of the society.

Historical Background

The very first inclusion of women in the Indian Army dates back to the year 1927 as Military Nursing Officers[2] during the British Raj. Thereafter, 1943 onwards, they were posted as Medical Officers in the British Indian Army specifically to look after the needs of fami-lies, public consisting of female populace and troops during their deployments[3]. After independence, since the year 1992, women of-

---

[1] The number of females in the Indian Armed Forces is alarmingly low, claims new report. (2020). Retrieved 14 October 2020, from https://www.timesnownews.com/mirror-now/society/article/females-women-ratio-indian-armed-forces-navy-air-force/207181

[2] Ministry of Defense Government of India, *Annual Report 2017-18*, pg. 13

[3] *Ibid.* pg. 14

ficers were inducted into the armed forces through 'Women Special Entry Scheme (WSES)'[4] after seeking approval from the Cabinet committee. Officers recruited under the WSE Scheme, in comparison to males who were recruited through the same scheme, were subjected to a shorter pre-commission period of training. They were recruited for a period of 5 years in streams like Corps of Signals, Corps of Engineers, Army Education Corps and Intelligence Corps. The WSES scheme got replaced by the SSC scheme in 2006 where the female officers were included later. Under it, they were recruited for a long period of 10 years which could be further extended by 4 years. However, the streams were still restricted and excluded Combat arms like armored corps and infantry. The Education and Legal corps were added to the list of streams in 2008 and 2020 saw women's induction as permanent commissioned officers in 8 more streams.

Women Empowerment through a Sociological Lens

Women empowerment is all about equipping and building women to decide the matters regarding their lives and employ those decisions in the actual physical space. The decision of the Supreme Court on permanent commission in Indian Army is a landmark judgment passed in the favor of empowered women who are braver than many and have joined the armed forces. This decision goes a long way to showcase that there are in fact no gender specific streams, and anyone who's fit and capable can be employed. This decision also breaks the dogmatic categorizations of gender socialization[5]. Gender stereotypes can be a result of gender socialization. From our childhood, we are taught how to walk, how to talk; we are taught what are the jobs that a man does and what are the jobs assigned to women. 'Gender' is a social identity[6]. We learn how to be a male and how to be a female in our society.

---

4 Women Officers in Indian Army | Entry Schemes Women. (2020). Retrieved 14 October 2020, from https://www.careerpathways.co.in/p/women-in-the-indian-army.html

5 Carter, M. (2014). Gender Socialization and Identity Theory. *Social Sciences, 3*(2), 242-263. doi: 10.3390/socsci3020242

6 McIntosh, M., & Butler, J. (1991). Gender Trouble: Feminism and the Subversion of Identity. *Feminist Review*, (38), 113.doi: 10.2307/1395391

The military has always been considered a profession unfit for women owing to the notion of gender roles, but induction of women in the Army has proved to be a huge step towards unlearning gender[7] empowerment of women. It would be unfair to say that women are made for only a certain category of jobs because they presently excel in almost every aspect of life and even perform better than men in some fields. Gender, therefore, is not at all an essential category in any sphere of employment.

The colonial discourse makes an inquiry into the Indian society by inviting views from different writers. One such view is that power is exercised socially and not just through institutions. It seeps into the social relationships. Therefore, when all the members of a society act in accordance with a single view point, the result is 'mindset'. So when we take up the issue of gender inequality we will have to go into the epistemology of the said issue.

Emmanuel Kant famously quoted, *'World is that which is experienced through glasses and which cannot be discarded'*[8]. It is not possible to change the basic biology of human beings to make them fit for a job but a job can be altered on the edges in order to fit in the pigeon holes of gender. It is true that the difference in genders cannot change but at the same time it doesn't mean that any person should be prevented from following their passions.

Bal Gangadhar Tilak has rightly said, *'Social reform has to be preceded by political reform'*[9]. It is seen many times that in order to prevent a commission or permit a commission, a law has to be made or a present law has to be amended. In order to empower women, making favorable laws and amending the unfavorable ones can be an appropriate step. An ideal has to be followed by the society in order to bring itself closer to being the ideal. We all know that 'social action' governs society. A social presentation of a person is nothing but how the society has been projected onto the person. The actions

---

[7] *ibid*

[8] Andreicut, D. (2014). Kant & Rand on Rationality & Reality. *Philosophy Now.*   Retrieved   from https://philosophynow.org/issues/101/Kant_and_Rand_on_Rationality_and_Reality

[9] Ghose, A. (1919). *Bal Gangadhar Tilak, his writings and speeches.* Madras: Ganesh & Co.

with their reactions give birth to problems such as gender inequality. Therefore, any action which can be categorized as women empowering has both positive and negative reactions. Therefore, when a law is placed, for example Dowry Prohibition Act 1961[10], the social reforms follow. The ideal, therefore, is set and now it is for the society to imbibe it and be governed by it. All such acts of women empowerment are met with a positive attitude from the society. Laws in favor of such acts transform the society. It brings a change in the thought process of the society. Women who were given a list of jobs are now bringing down gender barriers. It is advantage point of modernity. It is a way of truly becoming modern and not just developed.

Role of the Indian Judicial System in Women Empowerment

Permanent Commission in Armed Forces: Background
A Permanent Commission (PC) allows an officer to serve in the armed forces until one retires whereas the officers inducted through Short Selection Commission (SCC) serve for a period of 10 years which is extendable by a period of 4 more years. Women officers were not awarded PC in armed forces until recently, despite their long standing demands and efforts for the same. The Supreme Court, while delivering its verdict in the latest case granting women permanent commission in 10 streams of the army, reiterated that women empowerment is one of the most significant and powerful means for the prosperity and development of a nation.

The SC judgment came after a case was filed by 17 SCC women officers who even after the completion of 14 years in the service were not granted PC and were discharged unwillingly from the Indian Armed Forces[11]. They had in the court of law challenged a policy letter of 26th February 2008 issued by the Indian government which granted Permanent Commission to women SCC officers in all three divisions of the Military[12]. However, the letter was limited to just a

---

[10] Ministry Of Women & Child Development| GOI. (1961). *The Dowry Prohibition Act, 1961, (Act No. 28 of 1961).* India.

[11] *Lt. Cdr. Annie Nagaraj v Union of India.* [Writ Petition (C) No. 7336 of 20100]

[12] The Hindu. (2020). SC allows permanent commission for women in the Navy. Retrieved from https://www.thehindu.com/news/national/sc-allows-permanent-commission-for-women-in-navy/article31089114.ece

few categories only and was meant to function in accordance with future batches to be enrolled in SSC for their betterment. Before this, a case was instituted by the female officers in 2003 in the High Court of Delhi which attained a positive result in form of an order in the year 2010[13]. The order, however, was never implemented and was challenged by the government of India in the apex court. The Supreme Court in its present judgment upheld the ruling given by Delhi High Court in 2010 and issued directions to the central government to secure permanent commission and command posts for female officers in armed forces to ensure equality.

Indian Army: What Changed after Supreme Court's Judgment?
A woman officer, until now, under the SCC could only serve for a period of 14 years in the armed forces. She subsequently retired from the service. Pension was not an option for the female officers as 24 years of mandatory service was a prerequisite to obtain pension privileges. The apex court's judgment altered this condition and now the appointed female officers can serve up to the age of 60 years. Women in the armed forces are now subject to pension and other privileges. The appointed officer has the liberty to resign from the service any time before retirement at her own will. The woman officers serving the military under SSC can now opt for a permanent commission along with the pension privileges. As per the apex court, the amended policy decision will be applicable to all female officers who are presently serving under SSC.

Breaking Gender Stereotypes with Equality in Opportunities: A Constitutional Perspective

The apex court's judgment is a significant step towards the empowerment of women as it acknowledges that the physiological characteristics of a female do not bar her from getting equal entitlements under the Indian Constitution and the Indian army. It emphasizes the fact that there is a need to bring about a change in the mindset of men and public in general towards women in order to recognize the constitutional values of equality and rights. The commonly prevalent notion about there being a physiological difference between women and men is because of the deeply rooted gender stereotypi-

---

[13] *Union of India &Ors. v. Lt. Cdr. Annie Nagaraja & Ors.* SLP (C) Nos. 30791-96 of 2015

cal belief that women, being the *'weaker sex'*, won't be able to undertake tough tasks unlike their male counterparts. The apex court in its judgment rightly states that the center cannot keep denying women their rights by giving physiological and gender based excuses[14]. This change is based on women officer's right to equal opportunities which finds relevance in the constitution which prohibits discrimination on the grounds of sex[15] and grants equal opportunities of employment[16] to all the citizens. Article 14 also comes into play here which prescribes *"a right to rationality"*[17] forbidding any absolute or blanket prohibition. In the present case, it translates to the induction of women in the army.

Therefore, the burden to substantiate the distinction between men and women lies on the army itself, and such "differentiation has to be justified with reason"[18]. The state, judicial system and the civil society are obliged to internalize and successfully implement these rights in order to achieve gender justice in the armed forces which will grant women the same employment opportunities as men.

Shortcomings: Social and Political Dilemmas

Every woman who serves in the military faces problems of psychological, social and behavioral nature. It has been observed that most women are unsatisfied and uncomfortable with the atmosphere of the army profession. Women have a few issues of concern with the general environment of the army and these issues are omnipresent. Every country has faced its fair share of problems and limitations when the issue of women's acceptance into the army is brought up for consideration. Almost every nation state has had to fight the people with dogmatic-stereotypical nature who categorize this to be a useless agenda.

---

[14] Narasimhan, S. (2020). These Landmark Judgements Upholding the Dignity of Women by Indian Courts Will Make You Proud!. Retrieved 14 October 2020, from https://www.thebetterindia.com/38927/judgements-in-favour-of-gender-equality/
[15] The Constitution of India, 1950. Article 15(1)
[16] The Constitution of India, 1950. Article 15
[17] The Constitution of India, 1950. Article 14
[18] *ibid*

A large number of women officers feel that their competence, ability and credibility is not genuinely appreciated or recognized in the armed forces. Senior officers, in place of appreciating their recommendations, over-indulge themselves with the decision making process. Women in the army are often marginalized and are not invited to give opinions while taking serious decisions. In extreme cases, they have to work twice as hard as their male counterparts to get the recognition they deserve and prove themselves. Women, at all times, are more prone and vulnerable to scrutiny and criticism by the hands of men. It has been found that despite their technical and professional qualifications, women are often given menial and lower level jobs. Women also face the problems of social acceptance in the military among their male officers. If they showcase a feminine behavior, their acceptance declines amongst the male soldiers. Therefore, they are expected to behave and act in a more sturdy and manly way counteractive to their original nature.

A Global Overview of Women in Military

Unlike India, which initiated the induction of women in the army in early 90s, women around the world have been serving in the armies of their countries for a very long time now. The United States is considered as a trend setter with respect to the induction of women officers in the services. Almost 200,000 are presently serving in the armed forces of the US constituting 20% of its total strength[19]. They also participated in the Iraq operation in huge numbers. A lot changed for the US army during President Clinton's time. Women were finally permitted to serve as combat aircraft pilots and could also be assigned to serve on combat naval ships. Allowing them to serve in combat assignments opened up new avenues for them in the armed forces.

In UK, women serve on combat aircrafts, warships and fire artillery. The defense secretary of the UK has announced that anyone who is fit and willing should be allowed to combat[20]. Canada opened the

---

[19] Norville Valerie. *The Role of Women in Global Security.* United States Institute of Peace. https://www.usip.org/sites/default/files/SR264-The_role_of_Women_in_Global_Security.pdf

[20] The Guardian. (2014, May 8,). *Women set to get green light for combat roles in the British army.* https://www.theguardian.com/uk-news/2014/may/08/women-set-for-combat-roles-in-british-army

combat forces for women in 1989 and women have been serving in the combat roles since then in large numbers.

Norway was the first NATO[21] nation to permit women to serve in all combat roles in 1985. Germany increased the recruitment of women into the armed forces after 2001 when it permitted females to serve in the combat units. In South Africa, 21% of women make up the air force of the country. The governments around the world are slowly and gradually beginning to realize women's potential and most nations now allow them to serve in the artillery and combat roles.

Conclusion: A Way Forward

Women are now eligible for permanent commission in the Indian Armed Forces owing to the Supreme Court's latest decision in this direction, however, they have a long way to go before they get equal representation in the army. According to a report tabled in the Parliament in 2018, India's navy, air force and the army have a total of 3,653 women officers as compared to 62,507 male officers. India, being a developing country, cannot discriminate the recruitment process into armed forces on the basis of gender as that will hinder the socio-political and economic growth of the country and curtail the empowerment of women. Military units consisting of both women and men have coordinated well together and accomplished their missions in many insurgencies and battles. There is no proper rationale, whatsoever, for restricting women and prohibiting them from serving their nation at par with their male counterparts. To be efficient and optimally effective, armed forces require its most capable officers, irrespective of their gender.

There are many other nations which do not allow women to serve in the field/battle ground and engage in direct combat roles. In other countries, though allowed in the military, women never reach higher ranks despite being capable because of their gender. A nation cannot prosper if we leave women behind and think of moving forward with only men and their ideas. Women may be well equipped to discharge more traditional roles but the main argument here is that they should have the autonomy to choose. A woman should not

---

[21]Nielsen Vicki. *Women in uniform*. NATO Review. https://www.nato.int/nato-welcome/index.html

undertake a gender specific role by default and cultural expectations and traditional requirements shouldn't overshadow or limit her dreams. She, being a free individual, has every right to soar as high as she wants and if given freedom of choice, she holds the potential to conquer the world.

10

Role of Police and Women Empowerment

Priyanka Shekhar

Abstract

Police carries out a necessary role in preserving peace and justice in the society. The police stations majorly comprise of male police offices and women officers are nowhere to be seen. In many of the cases, women victims are unable to express their problem in front of a male officer, and they need a female police to assist them. A woman is empowered when she is given support to raise her voice against the injustice done to her and bring the police force in action. Also, to make the government policies more successful, women must enter the policing field. This study describes the crimes which are carried out against women along with the statistics of the crimes, major factors that cause these crimes, role a women police can play in policing, etc. Further, some suggestions have also been presented on the actionable steps that can be taken by the Indian government to enhance the strength of women, thus, helping in breaking the barriers and blazing a new path for women.

Crimes and Policing in India

Let us first get an understanding of what crime actually is. It is difficult to come to a particular definition of crime because of the changing notion of crime from place to place and time to time. We cannot ascertain what kind of human nature can be regarded as crime. Some jurists have attempted to defined crime as in their own way. Let's have a glance at few prominent definitions of crime:

According to **Prof. Kenny**; "crime are wrong whose sanction is positive and is in no way remissible by any private person but is remissible by Crown, if remissible at all." **Austin** posits that "A wrong which is pursued at the discretions of the injured party and his representatives is a civil injury; a wrong which is pursued by the sovereign or his subordinates is a crime." **John Gillin** gave a sociological definition of crime in the following terms: "Crime is an act that has been shown to be actually harmful to society, or that is believed to be socially harmful by a group of people that has the power to enforce its belief and that places such act under the ban of positive penalties." **Blackstone** in his "commentaries on the laws of England" has defined crime as "an act committed or omitted in violation of a public law either forbidding or commanding it". According to Blackstone, crime denotes an act which is in violation of public law. However, public Law has a broad meaning.

From the above definitions, it is clear that the definition of crime is not precise and exact. Till date, we do not have an exact and satisfactory definition of crime because it is not possible to define crime that would include act/omissions, that are considered to be criminal and at the same time exclude acts that are not criminal.

The concept of crime is subject to spatial, temporal and societal variations. Also, for a better understanding of what crime is, the three essentials can be considered:

- Crime is an act of commission or an act of omission on the part of a human being which is considered harmful by the State.
- The transgression of such harmful acts is prevented by a threat or sanction of punishment administered by the State; and
- The guilt of the accused is determined after the accusation against him has been investigated in legal proceedings of a special kind in accordance with the provision of law.

Crime Against Women

"To call woman the weaker sex is a libel; it is man's injustice to woman. If by strength is meant brute strength then indeed is woman less brute than man. If by strength is meant moral power then woman is immeasurably man's superior. Has she not greater intuition, is she not more self-sacrificing, has she not greater powers of endurance, has she not greater courage? Without her man could not be. If nonviolence is the law of our being the future is with woman. Who can make a more effective appeal to the heart than woman?" - Mahatma Gandhi

Crime against women is a burning topic in India. In a layman's language, crime against women is any direct or indirect physical or mental cruelty caused to a woman. Women are victims of all kinds of crime, be it murder, theft, cheating, etc., and yet there are crimes in which the victims are 'only women' and which are directly against them. These types of crimes are known as **"crimes against women"**.

Crime against women can be in any form depending upon the history, background, and culture, but one thing is certain that it causes great suffering to the women, their family as well the communities in which they live. This can be considered as a worldwide epidemic. Abuse against women is one of most severe and prevalent human rights abuse. It is rooted in gendered social systems rather than individual and spontaneous acts; it cuts through age, socio-economic, educational, and geographical boundaries; it affects all societies; and it is a major obstacle to overcoming gender inequality and discrimination globally. United Nation has defined Crime against women as *"any act of gender-based violence that results in, or is likely to result in, physical, sexual or psychological harm or suffering to women, including threats of such acts, coercion or arbitrary deprivation of liberty, whether occurring in public or in private life."* The UN Declaration on the Exclusion of Crime against Women (1993) states that "crime against women is an expression of traditionally imbalanced power relations between men and women, which have led to command over and discrimination against women by men and to the anticipation of the full development of women." Further, it states that "crime against women is one of the important social mechanisms by which women are forced into an outranked position associated with men."

Inter-caste marriages were forbidden in the Indian society and child marriage was common. Several progressive laws were enacted during the British rule, such as the Hindu Widows Remarriage Act, 1865 and the Brahmo Samaj Marriage Act, 1872. In the 19th century, the judiciary issued several landmark judgments to protest against dysfunctional customs and rituals, abolishing detestable practices such as Sati. After independence, Hindu Marriage Act, 1955 was passed, under which polygamy was abolished, minimum marriage age was set and remarriage in cases of spousal death or divorce was permitted. The Child Marriage (Restraint) Act, 1929 was abolished as it was not very effective and Prohibition of Child Marriage Act, 2006 came into force. In order to curb the sexual offences committees at workplace against women, the Sexual Harassment of Women at

Workplace (Prevention, Prohibition and Redressal) Act, 2013 was enacted. After the Nirbhaya casr, the government in passed the Criminal Amendment Act, 2013 or Anti-rape Law in order to impose strict penalties for rape and other sexual crimes. There are many other instances where women have experienced crime against them. In addition, numerous cases are not reported to the police to protect the family prestige.

The constitution has empowered the legislature to enact special laws for protecting women and many of them are in force. However, in spite of a plethora of special provisions and sections which give protection to the women not only outside but at home too, the crime rate is still rapidly increasing. We cannot generally notice any change in the men's brutality towards women! The increasing crime rate shows us that our education system and the laws need to be effective in changing the basic mentality and respect toward women.

Types of Crime and Statistical Analysis

Crime against women can be majorly classified into two categories i.e. Indian Penal Code and Special Local Laws. A total of 3,78,277 cases of crime against women (both IPC and SLL) were reported in India during the year 2018 as compared to 3,59,840 in the previous year. The crime rate with respect to crime against women was reported as 58.8 % in 2018.

The Crimes Identified in Indian Penal Code, 1860

Acid attacks (Sec 326A)
Cases reported - 131; crime rate - negligible
An extreme form of violence mostly perpetrated against women. It can be understood as an act of throwing an acid or any other corrosive substance done with an intention to torture, disfigure or kill. In India, a total of 131 cases have been reported in the year 2018, out of which 36 cases are from West Bengal.

Cruelty by husband or his relatives (Sec 498A)
Cases reported - 1,03,272; crime rate - 16.1%
Cruelty can be both mental and physical. It simply means doing an act which causes physical or mental harm to women's health

or body. These are generally carried out to harass her so that the unlawful demands of the husband or his relatives can be fulfilled. These practices have been very old, however, a shocking number of 1,03,272 cases have been reported in the year 2018. West Bengal (16,951) had the highest number of cases followed by Uttar Pradesh (14,233), Rajasthan (12,250) and Assam (11,261). Delhi reported 3,416 cases.

Importation of girls from a foreign country (up to 21 years of age) (Sec. 366 B IPC)
Cases reported - 4; crime rate - negligible
A decline has been observed in cases registered under this crime head in 2018 over 2017 (5 cases). Manipur, Telangana, Madhya Pradesh and West Bengal each had 1 cases recorded.

Kidnapping & abduction of women (Sec 363-373)
Cases reported - 6,051; crime rate - 0.9%
Kidnapping and abduction is defined under section 336 of IPC. Kidnapping and abduction are carried out in order to murder the women (Sec 364) or for ransom (Sec 364A) or in order to compel her for marriage (Sec 366). In India, a total of 6051 cases have been reported in 2018.Out of 6051 cases, about 1,537 cases have been reported from Rajasthan, whereas states such as Nagaland and Sikkim had 0 cases! Delhi reported 223 cases.

Dowry deaths (Sec 304B)
Cases reported - 5,266; crime rate - 0.8%
Dowry is basically giving of property, money or goods by the bride's family to the groom's family. It is the main reason for discrimination towards women in India. In spite of the Dowry Prohibition Act, 1961, there are educated people who proudly display the articles of dowry in the marriage as the status symbol. Out of 5,266 cases that have been reported in India in the year 2018, Madhya Pradesh has been recorded with the highest number of 881 cases.

Molestation (Sec 354)
Cases reported - 89,097; crime rate - 13.8%
Molestation also known as sexual abuse, which includes touching of private parts, taking pornographic pictures or videos, etc. 89,097 cases have been reported in 2018 in India. The highest

number of cases have been reported in Uttar Pradesh (12,555) followed by Maharashtra (10,835) and Odisha (9,973). Delhi recorded 2,705 cases in the same year.

Rape (Sec 375)
Cases reported - 33,356; crime rate - 5.2%
Rape is the fastest growing crime in India. A total of 33,356 cases have been registered during the year 2018. 13.8% (5,433 out of 33,356) cases were reported in Madhya Pradesh, followed by Rajasthan (4,335), Uttar Pradesh (3,946) and Maharashtra (2,142). Delhi reported 1215 cases.

Further 4,097 cases of attempt to commit rape have been recorded in 2018 which includes both women (18 years and above) and girls (18 years and below). Highest number of cases have been recorded in West Bengal (944), followed by Uttar Pradesh (661) and Rajasthan (620).

Crimes Identified under Special and Local Laws

Dowry Prohibition Act, 1961
Crime recorded - 12,826; crime rate - 2%
The cases registered under Dowry Prohibition Act have increase by 0.4 % as compared to the year 2017 (10,189). Maximum cases were reported in Uttar Pradesh (4,371), followed by Bihar (2,094) and Odisha (1,595).

Indecent Representation of Women (Prohibition) Act, 1986
Cases reported - 22; crime rate - negligible
Rajasthan reported 7 cases out of 22 in the year 2018.

Commission of Sati Prevention Act, 1987
Like previous years, no case was registered under the Commission of Sati Prevention Act across the country during the year 2018.

The Immoral Traffic (Prevention) Act, 1956
Cases reported - 1,459; crime rate - 0.2%
The cases herein refers only to women victims. This includes **A)** procuring, inducing children, for the sake of prostitution (Section 5), **B)** detaining a person in premises where prostitution is carried on (Section 6), **C)** prostitution in or in the vicinity of

public places (Section 7), **D)** seducing or soliciting for purpose of prostitution (Section 8) and **E)** Other Sections under ITP Act. The highest number of cases were reported in Tamil Nadu (386), followed by Maharashtra (200) and Karnataka (179).

Further, out of 1459 cases that have been reported under Immoral Traffic (Prevention) Act, 253 cases have been registered under Section 5 (procuring, inducing children, for the sake of prostitution), 143 under Section 6 (detaining a person in premises where prostitution is carried on), 172 under section 7 (prostitution in or in the vicinity of public places), 120 under section 8 (seducing or soliciting for purpose of prostitution) and the rest 771 in other sections of Immoral Traffic Act.

The Protection of Women from Domestic Violence Act, 2005

Cases recorded - 579; crime rate - 0.1%

A total of 579 cases were recorded in 2018 as compared to 614 in 2017. The maximum number of cases were recorded in Madhya Pradesh (275), followed by Kerala, where 175 cases were recorded. Delhi (2) had a decline in the number of cases as compared with the previous year (6).

Cyber Crimes/Information Technology Act, 2000

Cases recorded - 1244; crime rate - 0.1%

Out of 1244 cases, 862 were recorded under publishing or transmitting of sexually explicit material (Sec 67A/67B (Girls) IT Act), and 382 were recorded under other women centric cybercrimes (ex. blackmailing/defamation/fake profile). Assam (184) had the highest number of cases in cybercrimes whereas Arunachal Pradesh and Mizoram recorded 0 cases.

Disposal of Cases Reported Under Crime Against Women

Out of total of 4,76,586 cases pending in 2018 under Indian Penal Code, 3,16,692 cases have been disposed off by the police while the rest were pending for the year 2019. For the 5,54,936 cases pending under SLL in 2018, 34.3% were pending for 2019.

The following are the statistics related to the disposal of the cases by the courts.

For the crimes that have been defined under IPC:
* **Total cases for trial - 14,22,587**
* Cases pending trial from the previous year - 11,86,156
* Cases sent for trial during the year - 2,36,431
* Cases disposed off without trial - 18,928
* Cases in which trial was completed - 1,13,483
* Cases disposed off by the court - 1,32,411
* **Cases pending trial at the end of the year - 12,90,176**
* Conviction rate - 21.9%

For the crimes that have been defined under SLL:
* **Total cases for trial - 15,98,471**
* Cases pending trial from the previous year - 13,15,493
* Cases sent for trial during the year - 2,82,978
* Cases disposed off without trial - 19,713
* Cases in which trial was completed - 15,502
* Cases disposed off by the court - 16,287
* **Cases pending trial at the end of the year - 11,59,597**
* Conviction rate - 32.1%

It can be clearly seen from the above figures that the legal resolution has been getting delayed in the matters of crimes against women. Many cases are pending at the end of the year, and many are being disposed off without trials. This is surely not a good precedent.

Factors Leading to Crime Against Women

Social, physical, cultural, biological and legal factors are the root cause for the growing crimes against women. One of the major reasons for commission of this crimes is lack of education. Other causes of crime against women are as follows:

Societal causes: Man holds a superior status as per the Indian society and the women is merely his companion. A woman is never regarded as a person in her own right. She is, first the daughter, then the wife and lastly the mother of a child. Many men are deliberately trained to be aggressive and strong to retain their dominance whereas a woman is always taught to be passive and compliant.

Psychological causes: The narrow-mindset does not allow an equal power to the women in many families. It is a common belief that the most significant task of women is to take care of the husband and family. She should do the work, whenever the conditions require financial assistance, but if her work causes inconvenience to the family, she should quit the job. She should never forget her domestic role even though she is educated and employed. She is not allowed to mix easily with men while she works. We do see people concerned for women safety, security and empowerment but the reality is that they don't like to see the women becoming independent.

Unemployment or Under-employment: Occasionally, some men have been observed to put the blame for their failure on their wives, which leads to crime against them out of frustration. There are instances where husbands have even left their wives despite the fact that the wives are earning to support the entire family. Sitting without a job at home, many narrow-minded men imagine being mocked by the wife. As a result, unemployed men have been found beating their wives on very trivial domestic matters.

Alcohol: One of the main reasons of crimes against women is alcohol. Alcohol has a significant impact on the mind and body. Excessive consumption can lead to repercussions like loss of property, dicord between husband and wife, quarrels with the family members, cruelty, beating, etc.

Marital maladjustment: Marital maladjustment is a clash between the husband and wife over issues that are related to thinking, working, dressing up, behavior and adjustment with the family.

Women in Policing

"Empowered women who reach tough or unconventional positions make choices not sacrifices" - IPS Kiran Bedi

According to "Status of Policing in India Report, 2019" there are only 7.28% women in Indian police force and out of these women, 90% are constables while less than 1% hold supervisory positions. These are very disturbing numbers.

In 2013, the Ministry of Home Affairs reiterated the goal of 33% preservation for women in police and recommended that at least three female sub-inspectors and ten female constables be employed at each police station to ensure that female aid services are available at all times. In spite of reservations and advertisement for vacancies, the seats are not filled. In some states, the women do not match the employability category, while there are not enough takers for the job in other states.

In 2015, the central government proposed the establishment of Investigation Units for Crimes against Women (IUCAW) at police stations in crime-prone districts across states. These units shall have 15 specialist investigators dealing exclusively with crimes against women. At least one third of the investigating personnel is expected to be females.

However, the question is what is the utility of women in policing? The police service must be inclusive of all parts of the society in which it works. Sex, race and faith diversity would ensure that a single segment of the population does not control the police service. This guarantees not only fair employment conditions, but also greater access to justice for women and children in particular.

According to a United Nations Women Report in 2011-12 titled "Progress of the World's Women: In Pursuit of Justice", the presence of a women police officer has a positive connection to incidents of sexual harassment, and that women empowerment is a major component of the justice system centered on gender issues. The report also stated that it could be difficult for women to approach male police officers. In fact, men and women who suffered from sexual harassment tended to report to women police.

A plus point that is stated by the "Status of Policing 2019 Report" is that Police women are less likely to use excessive violence, and other police officers may decrease their use of force in their presence. Also, in a study from 2010 it was observed that ""*twenty years of exhaustive research demonstrates that women police officers utilise a style of policing that relies less on physical force, and more on communication skills that defuse potentially violent situations. Women police officers are therefore much less likely to be involved in occurrences of police brutality, and are also much more likely to effectively respond to police calls regarding violence against women.*"

Ministry of Home Affairs circular in 2015 has rightly stated that the legislations on crime against women are not yielding fruitful result due to the skewed ratio of women in police. So, what are the factors that stop a women to enter into this occupation? Firstly, there is a strong belief that fighting is, by its nature, a male occupation; that the police force is a male jurisdiction and, thus, inappropriate for the physique and temperament of women. Secondly, most women tend not to apply because they believe that this is not suitable job for them or due to family who are against such career or the work timing is unsuitable for them or due to the gender discrimination or the sexual harassment that they have to face, etc. Thirdly, due to the harassment from their male colleagues, many women stay away from this profession.

Thus, it can be concluded that recruitment and promotion of women police officers is necessary to increase the representation of women at various levels. The following are the ways in which we can empower the women and increase the women police officers:

- In order to increase the number of police women at all levels, states should make commitments to ensure an equal balance between men and women.
- A common and combined post must be created and clear targets must be assigned for the number of women which need to be recruited in every recruitment year at all levels.
- Regular gender sensitization training for the police will also help counteract patriarchal attitudes.
- Departments should partner with local media and educational organisations to publicise opportunities for women in the police.
- Regular seminars, webinars and workshops should be conducted by the lawyers, government officials, and NGO's to create awareness about the role of women in police.
- State governments should focus on making the institutions gender-friendly and developing facilities that cater to the needs and responsibilities of women which includes the establishment of crèches, elimination of sexual abuse at the workplace and construction of separate toilets.
- Women's role is not restricted to answering calls or making entries in diary. The government and the police departments must ensure that they are being given same opportunities as the men.

- Any government that comes to power must build a level playing field to open up opportunities and meet the needs of diverse parts of society.
- Also, All Women Run Police Stations must be set up in every state.
- It must be remembered that the police needs women for the ideals and efficiency they have and not the other way round! Barak Obama has rightly said "Lifting women up lifts up our economy and lifts up our country... We've got to make sure that... Somebody is standing up for them".

References

Criminology and Penology (3rd edn; New York) In soviet Russia crime has been defined in terms of socially dangerous acts. Sec. 6 of R.S.F.S.R. Code of 1926.

Government of India, Ministry of Home Affairs, Advisory (2013), D.O.No.15011/21   SC/ST   – W:https://mha.gov.in/sites/default/files/AdvisoryWomenPolice-290513.pdf

Government of India, Ministry of Home Affairs, Advisory (2015), 15011/72/2014   –   SC/ST   – W: https://mha.gov.in/sites/default/files/CrimesagainstWomen06 01.PDF

Government of India, Ministry of Home Affairs, National Crime Record Bureau, Crime in India, 2018, https://ncrb.gov.in/en/crime-india-2018

Government of India, Ministry of Home Affairs, National Crime Record Bureau, Crime in India, 2017, https://ncrb.gov.in/en/crime-india-2017

Murthy H.V., Sreenivasa. History of India Part-I. Luckhnow: Eastern Book Company, (2006) Apte Prabha, Women in Indian Society. New Delhi: Concordia Publishing House, (1996) 15.

NCRB, (2018), Crime in India: Statistics-2011, National Crime Records Bureau, Ministry of Home Affairs, Government of India, New Delhi

UN Women (2011-12), Progress of the World's Women: In Pursuit of Justice, p. 59

National Centre for Women and Policing, Retrieved from http://womenandpolicing.com

Crime against women, Retrieved from https://ncrb.gov.in/sites/default/files/crime_in_india_table_additio nal_table_chapter_reports/Chapter%205-15.11.16_2015.pdf

Facts and figures: Ending violence against women (November 2019), Retrieved from https://www.unwomen.org/en/what-we-do/ending-violence-against-women/facts-and-figures

The Role of Women in Policing Today, Retrieved from https://www.joineps.ca/AboutEPS/Women%20in%20Policing/The Role

Nithya Subramanian (Sep 21, 2019), *In charts: Only 7% of India's police force is women. This hurts investigations into gender violence,* https://scroll.in/article/937265/in-charts-only-7-of-indias-police-force-is-women-this-hurts-investigations-into-gender-violence

Pavani Nagaraja Bhat, *Women in Police: India needs more than just tokenism by political parties,* https://www.humanrightsinitiative.org/blog/women-in-police-india-needs-more-than-just-political-promises-to-raise-numbers

11

Women Empowerment and Welfare: The Indian Context

Jatinder Singh

Abstract

This chapter explains the current status of women empowerment in India. Women empowerment in the present times is a core issue of the 21st century but it is still an illusion of reality. In our day to day life, we observe the brutality and rough treatment women face in the society. Women empowerment is a vital instrument to bring women to the mainstream by exploring the possibilities and making resources available to them. A comparative study of NFHS-3 and NFHS-4 has been made with the help of statistical data. Various welfare schemes and legislative measures undertaken by the government of India for the betterment of women are also discussed. Status of India is also checked under Women, Peace and Security Index (WPS) within the states and among the neighboring countries. It is quite pertinent to mention that there is a transformation in the Indian traditional way of thinking slowly and steadily. Women are slowly being given chance in every sphere of life at par with their counterparts, but it is still a long way to provide the women self-respect and dignity, along with favorable environment so that they excel in their lives and ultimately contribute in the prosperity of the nation.

Introduction

All around the world, women, men, boys and girls suffer manifold problems in the form of vulnerability and violence that directly impact their security, development and well-being in day-to-day life. Conflicts results in destructive consequences for everyone, but women and girls are the real victims. Generally, women and girls have low access to resources to protect and sustain themselves, are mainly the intentional target of gender-related violence and are more often excluded from the mainstream participations essential for their peace and security (Oxfam.org). There has been a holistic and comprehensive approach over the years to formulate and implement multiple   policies and programmes to acknowledge and address these realities. Despite this, the gender based violence is prevailing and women are the most likely target. In the present times, focus on gender equality and empowerment of women in all walks of life are vital for achieving socially, economically and ecologically sustainable development in the world. Development is a precondition for peace and without the mass inclusion of all sections of the society, such as marginalized and non-marginalized, deprived and helpless, etc., it is not possible to achieve such goals. We can imagine a progressively more peaceful and prospective world only with the equal involvement of women in every nook and corner of the society. In 2000, the UN Security Council adopted Resolution (UNSCR) 1325 on "Women, Peace and Security" that acknowledges the lopsided effects of war and conflict on women. On the contrary, it also emphasizes the role of women in prevention and resolution of the conflicts, as well as in peace and reconstruction processes. It goals at enhancing women's role in decision-making capacities with regard to conflict prevention, resolution and peace building.

Women Empowerment and Protection

The concept of gender equality is well described in the Constitution of India. It grants a special privilege to women in every walk of life at par with the men. States are directed to adopt measures and policies in the favor of women to bring them into the mainstream of life. Constitution has special provisions to eradicate cumulative socio-economic and political disadvantages faced by women. The women have been enriched with fundamental rights so as not to be discriminated on the basis of biological and physical differences and have equal safeguard under the ambit of the law. It also imposes a fundamental duty on the part of the citizens to uproot the offensive practices that hamper women's dignity.

Women empowerment is a process that gives women the equal opportunities in economic, cultural, social and political spheres of life and realise their full potential. This can only be possible by giving freedom to women in their decision making at home and outside. The Ministry of Women and Child Development has taken numerous initiatives to empower women and to ensure their safety and security. Women empowerment in India profoundly depends upon a wide range of variables, including geographical locations (urban/rural), status of education, social status (caste and class), and age. Policies and legislations exist at every level in almost every sector of the economy to address the gender based discrimination and ensure equal participation of women in every sphere of life. However, there are loopholes in practical application of policies at the ground level. The key factor behind this gap is the patriarchal setup that rules the societies at large. As such, women and girls are restricted to homes, have less or no access to education, health facilities, decision-making, , etc., and experience higher rates of violence. Some of the indicators and measures of women empowerment are discussed below.

Table 1. Women empowerment and gender based violence (age 15-49 years; in percent)

Indicators	2005-06	2015-16
Currently married women who usually participate in household decisions	76.5	84
Women who worked in the last 12 months and were paid in cash	28.6	24.6
Ever-married women who have ever experienced spousal violence	37.2	31.1
Ever-married women who have experienced violence during any pregnancy	na	3.9
Women owning a house and/or land (alone or jointly with others)	15.1	53.0
Women having a mobile phone that they themselves use	na	45.9
Women aged 15-24 years who use hygienic methods of protection during their menstrual period	na	57.6

Source: NFHS-3, NFHS-4; na: not applicable

NFHS-4 shows an improvement in the overall upliftment of women in India. Between the time periods 2005–06 and 2015–16, the per-centage of currently married women who usually participate in household decisions has increased by 7 percent. There is a decline in the payments to working women in cash by 4 percent since NFHS-3. A small decrease in the proportion of ever-married women aged 15-49 years reporting spousal physical or sexual violence is observed n NFHS-4. Spousal brutality decreased by 6 percentage points, from 37.2 percent to 31.1 percent at the national level and 4 percent women faced some sorts of cruelty in the family during pregnancy as per NFHS-4. A considerable threefold increment in the percentage of assets ownership (alone or jointly) during the NFHS-4 among women is noticed i.e. 38 percent. Women have got ownership rights more rapidly due to both government interventions and spread of education. Use of mobile phone themselves is also an indication of accelerated literacy and education among women. Drastic change is recorded among the women of 15-24 years age regarding their menstrual health and hygiene in the span of 10 years which tallies at 57.6 percent, as given in NFHS-4. In a nutshell, there is a considerable improvement in the different aspects of women since 2005-06.

Table 2. Employment status of women aged 15-49 for the period of 12 months before survey

Indicators	2005-06 (in %)	2015-16 (in %)
Residence		
Urban	29.3	24.9
Rural	49.4	33.3
Age (in years)		
15-19	33.4	18.5
20-29	38.5	25
30-39	50.6	37.4
40-49	49.7	39.1

Source: NFHS-3, NFHS-4

Among the women of age group 15-49, the status of employment both in terms of age and residence has been taken into consideration. In 2005-06, there were 29.3 percent women in the urban areas of India who were employed and almost 50 percent were employed in the rural areas. On the other hand, during NFHS-4, a slow decline was observed in the employment status of women. There were 25 percent employed women in the urban areas in 2015-16 and the rural women employment was 33 percent. Thus, there is overall decline in the employment of women since 2005-06. In the age group 15-19, a highest decline in employment was observed. The decline was the lowest in the age group 40-49.

Table 3. Women's cash earnings compared with their husband's cash earnings (in percent)

Age (in years)	More		Less		Same	
	2005-06	2015-16	2005-06	2015-16	2005-06	2015-16

15-19	7.3	15.7	79.8	59.6	6.0	19.4
20-24	6.8	18.4	79.8	55.6	8.8	21.6
25-29	8.0	17.5	79.0	53.9	8.8	24.1
30-39	10.8	19.5	72.5	53.6	11.1	22.5
40-49	12.6	20.2	66.8	51.1	12.5	24.2

Source: NFHS-3, NFHS-4

This table exclusively depicts the earnings of women in contrast to their husband's earnings that signifies the self-dependency of women. In terms of different age groups, it was found that there has been an increased cash earnings of women irrespective of their age groups in 2015-16 as compared to their husbands. In the age group of 40-49, 20.2 % women had higher earnings than men. Further, there was a decrease in the number of women earning less with respect to their husbands. There were only 24.2 percent women who had same earnings to that of their husbands in 2015-16 which was only 12.5 percent in 2005-06.

Table 4. Freedom of movement to women

Place	Years	
	2005-06 (in %)	**2015-16 (in %)**
Alone to the market	51.4	54.2
Alone to the health facility	47.7	50
Alone to places outside the village/community	37.7	48
Alone to all three places	33.5	40.5

Source: NFHS-3, NFHS-4

In terms of allowing women to move freely without family indulgence, there was not a significant change in moving alone among women. Under NFHS-4, the percentage rose from 51.4 to 54.2 only. Similarly to visit doctor and other health facilities, there was an increment of 2.3 percent. Further, an almost 10 percent increase in the percentage of women visiting the places outside their villages and communities was observed. There were 33.5 percent women who visited all of these places alone in 2005-06, and the percentage rose to 40.5 in 2015-16.

Figure 1. Percentage of women aged 15-19 exposed to media

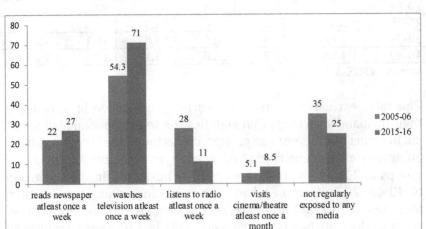

Source: NFHS-3, NFHS-4

Exposure to media is also one of the measures of women empowerment. The trend of listening to radio has gone down over the years among Indian women. There is an increase in the habit of reading newspaper and watching television at least once a week. There is no substantial rise in the visits to the cinema theatres by women since NFHS-3 (3.4 percent increase only). There is also a 10 percent decline in the number of women not regularly exposed to any media.

Table 5. Access to money and credit in percent

	Access to money			
Schooling	Have money that they can decide how to use		Have bank or savings account that they themselves use	
	2005-06	2015-16	2005-06	2015-16
Up to 5 years	37.9	41.8	10.9	43
5-7 years	41.1	40.2	12.1	45.5
8-9 years	41.1	38	15.1	49.2
10-11 years	48.1	39.2	22.3	56.8
12 or more years	59.7	50.1	40.9	72.4

Source: NFHS-3, NFHS-4

An important indicator of women's empowerment is whether women have a bank account or a savings account that they themselves use and their choice of using money at their own will. Classification of women's access to money and credit has been made in terms of schooling years. With the increasing schooling years of women, there is a considerable increase in the bank accounts operated by women themselves. The opening of bank accounts has increased significantly since NFHS-3. It is also seen that with the increase in schooling years, less number of women decide to spend their money as per their wish. The proportion of such women is noted to significantly fall in the category of more than ten years of schooling.

Table 6. Women knowledge and use of microcredit programmes (in percent)

Age (in years)	Have knowledge of a microcredit programme		Have taken a loan from a microcredit programme	
	2005-06	2015-16	2005-06	2015-16
15-19	30.8	31.7	0.8	1.1
20-24	37.5	38.6	2.5	3.8
25-29	40.3	42.6	4.4	7.9
30-39	41.4	44	6	11.2
40-49	42.4	44.7	5.9	11.8

Source: NFHS-3, NFHS-4

With age, women are observed to become more knowledgeable about the microcredit programmes. There were 44.7 percent women having such knowledge in 2015-16, as compared to 42.4 percent women possessing such knowledge under NFHS-3. Also, maximum percentage of women in the age group of 30-39 and 40-49 years have taken loan from a microcredit programme. In the lower age groups, no significant difference in knowledge among women was seen under NFHS-3 and NFHS-4.

Women, Peace and Security Index (WPS)

The Women, Peace and Security Index has a revolutionary and a transformative potential. It is an influential factor in democratic decision-making, moving from gender inequality to equality and from conflict and violence to sustainability and blissful world. The agenda has now got worldwide recognition, but deep rooted evils prevalent since long like patriarchy, inequalities, militarized masculinities and discriminatory habits are the major impediments that hinder the effective implementation. There is a dire need for a significant trans-formation and put thoughts into action. Different agencies and governments, the United Nations, civil society, private sector and other actors must work for strengthening women. To ensure the gender perspective as well as women's participation, protection and rights are important in peacekeeping, policy-making and reconstruction.

The WPS Index is a straightforward and a crystal clear measure that particularly deals with the women's autonomy and empowerment at their homes, in the community, and in the society. The index takes into consideration the three basic dimensions that focus upon the well-being of women: inclusion (economic, social, and political); justice (formal laws and informal discrimination); and security (at the individual, community, and societal levels). The index reveals a wide range of performances around the globe. The overall rankings display the status of women in different countries throughout the globe, ranging from 0.904 at the top (Norway) to .351 at the bottom (Yemen).

There are profound commonalities and adversities across and within the regions that indicate the scope for the countries to improve to become par with their high ranked countries. Inter-regional differences are observed to be significant. For illustration, in Central and Eastern Europe and Central Asia, Estonia ranks 12th and Azerbaijan ranks 123rd. Same is the case with Latin America and the Caribbean, between Trinidad and Tobago, at 41, and Haiti, at 140.

The Indian Context

With more than 1.3 billion people, India's subcontinent is widely sparse in size, income, human development, and in terms of women inclusion, justice, and security. In India, top-performers are con-densed in the southern part of the subcontinent, while the worst performing regions rangesfrom Rajasthan to Assam on the northern side. A study conducted by the Hindustan Times found similar geographic patterns in their "Women Empowerment Index". McKinsey Global Institute's Index has also found Mizoram, Kerala, and Goa as the best performing states in this respect. Kerala, being the topper on the sub-national index, secured second for women education and first for cell phone use. Kerala's high ranking under security sub-index reveals minimal organized violence and intimate partner violence, but shows contrasting crime rates. In the state of Manipur, schooling, employment rates and participation in household decision-making are comparatively higher than the rest of the country. However, there are major differences among the security indicators where the state performs poorly. Manipur records the highest rates of intimate partner violence and son bias, and ranks second in battle deaths (organized violence). The state has been widely known for ethnic conflict, which is associated with physical, emotional, and sexual violence against women, who have been used as a weapon of patriarchal wars and discrimination (Singha, 2017). Manipur ranks at the bottom on the sub-national index in India. There are also some good ranking states that perform very poorly in other areas. For example, Karnataka ranks 4th overall but 20th on the inclusion sub-index. The UT of Chandigarh is on the top on the inclusion sub-index but 18th on justice and 16th on security. Likewise, Meghalaya lags very behind on the sub-national index (Gneezy, Leonard, and List 2009). The average performance reflects the fact that the main Khasi community comprises only half the population and the index does not include sub-national laws such as legislation on succession (Nongbri 1988).

The WPS index comprises of some dimensions and indicators that are discussed in the detailed form as below.

Dimensions and Indicators	Definition
	Inclusion
Education	Average years of women education ages 25 and more
Employment	Proportion of women 25 and above years old and are employed
Cell phone use	Percentage of women of age 15 and above who report having mobile phone and use it for receiving and making personal calls
Financial Inclusion	Percentage of women having age 15 and above reported operating an individual or joint account at some bank or use online money service
Parliamentary Representation	Percentage of seats reserved for women in both the houses of the Parliament of India
	Justice
Legal Discrimina-	Cumulative score for the set of rules that border the

tion	ability of women ability to partake in the community and nation or that distinguish between men and women
Son Bias	The extent to which the ratio of the number of boys born to the number of girls born surpass the normal demographic rate of 1.05
Discriminatory Norms	Proportion of men aged 15 years and more who disagree with the statement: "It is perfectly acceptable for any woman in your family to have a paid job outside the home if she wants one"
	Security
Intimate Partner Violence	Proportion of women who face physical or sexual violence committed by their intimate partner in the previous 12 months
Community Safety	Percentage of women ages 15 and older reporting that they "feel safe walking alone at night in the city or area where you live"
Organized Violence	Yearly average number of battle causalities due to state-based, nonstate, and one-sided conflicts per 100,000 people between 2016 and 2018

Source: GIWPS, 2019

Table 7. WPS Indicators of top 10 states of India

State	Rank	Index Score	Mean years of schooling	Financial inclusion (%)	Employment (%) among	Cellphone use (%)	Parliamen tary (%)	Females who participate in	Sex ratio - at birth	% females allowed to work if suitable jobs	Lifetime Intimate Partner Violence (%)	Organized violence
Kerala	1	0.652	9.88	70.60	25.97	81.20	5.00	92.10	1.05	40.76	14.30	0.04
Mizoram	2	0.621	7.36	57.40	53.74	77.30	0.10	96.00	1.03	14.29	17.00	1.64
Tamil Nadu	3	0.592	6.38	77.00	42.87	62.00	10.26	84.00	1.22	33.68	40.60	0.11
Karnataka	4	0.589	5.02	59.40	44.97	47.10	4.00	80.40	1.12	30.58	20.50	0.16
Chandigarh	5	0.567	9.31	79.60	22.52	74.20	50.00	96.60	1.11	77.78	22.50	3.70
Gujarat	6	0.555	5.22	48.6	33.60	47.9	19.23	85.4	1.13	39.20	20.1	1.93
Maharashtra	7	0.554	6.50	45.30	43.38	45.60	12.50	89.30	1.13	49.22	21.40	0.90
West Bengal	8	0.554	5.48	43.50	25.95	41.80	30.95	89.90	1.09	65.09	32.80	0.69
Andhra Pradesh	9	0.547	4.03	66.30	50.58	36.20	8.00	79.90	1.03	40.55	43.20	2.34
Himachal Pradesh	10	0.546	6.83	68.80	59.83	73.90	0.10	90.80	1.11	81.39	5.90	0.58

Here an attempt has been made to look at the top ten states and UTs of India in terms of WPS rankings and performance under various indicators of WPS Index. Kerala is first in the overall rankings of WPS in India. It also leads in the years of schooling, while Andhra Pradesh is at the last, i.e., 4.03 years. In Chandigarh, women have opened more bank accounts and use online money services as well. In addition, in Tamil Nadu and Kerala, there is also a considerable financial inclusion which is 77 percent and 70.6 percent, respectively. West Bengal has the lowest financial inclusion among these states. In terms of employment among women aged 15-49, Himachal Pradesh tops the ranking while Chandigarh is the last. Use of cell phone among women is most prevalent in Kerala, while cell phones are used by women the least in Andhra Pradesh. Although Kerala has high literacy rate, but Chandigarh and west Bengal offer the parliamentary representation to women the most. In Himachal Pradesh, women get the least reservation in the Parliament. Decision making power is vested significantly high in all states and UTs. However, in Chandigarh and Mizoram, women make use of their decisions making powers in their family affairs the most. Sex-ratio at birth is almost the same in all states and UTs. In Chandigarh and Himachal Pradesh, women are allowed to do jobs outside homes by their family members, but jobs to women are highly restricted in Mizoram. Only 14.29 percent women work to earn for their families. In Andhra Pradesh, women face the maximum brutalities either in their homes or outside, whereas the rate of violence is found to be least in Himachal Pradesh. A big concern is that well planned offences are carried out against women in Chandigarh, which is a serious concern.

Table 8. WPS Index of India and its neighboring countries

Country	WPS Value	INCLUSION				JUSTICE			SECURITY		
		Education	Financial Inclusion	Employment	Cellphone Use	Parliamentary Representation	Legal Discrimination	Son Bias	Discriminatory Work Norms	Intimate Partner Violence	Community Safety	Organised Violence
Nepal	0.71	3.6	41.6	83.4	81.6	33.5	32	1.07	18	11.2	49.8	0.00

Sri Lanka	0.68	10.3	73.4	37.2	70.0	5.3	27	1.04	33	18.4	54.1	0.00
Maldives	0.67	6.2	65.4	40.7	71.4	4.7	18	1.07	33	5.6	63.1	0.00
Bhutan	0.66	1.7	27.7	66.2	71.4	15.3	16	1.04	33	6.1	61.7	0.00
India	**0.63**	**4.8**	**76.6**	**26.5**	**74.9**	**12.2**	**23**	**1.11**	**25**	**22.0**	**64.0**	**0.06**
Bangladesh	0.61	5.4	35.8	37.8	73.1	20.6	34	1.05	57	26.9	69.9	0.03
Pakistan	0.46	3.7	7.0	24.2	34.0	20.0	38	1.09	73	14.5	63.2	0.43
Afghanistan	0.37	1.9	7.2	51.6	46.2	27.3	40	1.06	51	46.1	12.2	63.63

Source: GIWPS, 2019

In this table, a comparative study of India and its neighboring countries is carried out with respect to the indicators of WPS Index. India ranks fifth in WPS score, whereas Nepal performs the best and Afghanistan performs very poorly. There are three main indicators, i.e., inclusion, justice and security, which are further sub-divided into more categories. Under inclusion, there is education, financial inclusion, employment, cellphone use and parliamentary representation. Justice is sub-categorized into legal discrimination, son bias, discriminatory work norms and intimate partner violence, while security has community safety and organized violence as the main measures. In Sri Lanka, there is a more than 10 years of average schooling for women aged 25 years and more. In Bhutan and Afghanistan, the average schooling is just 2 years which is a dilapidated condition. There is a large chunk of women having their bank accounts and operated by themselves which reflects a large extent of financial inclusion, but this percentage is the least in Afghanistan and Pakistan. In Nepal, 83.4 percent women of age 25 years and above are employed, which is quite a good signal for the Nepalese economy, whereas India marks the least at 26.5 percent. Nepalese women make use of cellphones the most, while in Afghanistan and Pakistan, the proportion is 46.2 percent and 34 percent respectively. Representation of women in political affairs is also rich in Nepal, while they are given the least representation in Sri Lanka and Maldives. In Nepal, women face the least discrimination and son bias. India is a big victim of son bias, as represented by the sex ratio imbalance. In many countries in the list, the men allow women to work to a large extent. In Afghanistan, there is a widespread organized violence against women at a significant rate of 63.6 percent, which is alarming and concerning. No other country has such severe condition.

Legislative Framework for Protection of Women in India

On the legal front, the concerned ministry is active in ensuring the protection of the vulnerable women. There are different laws that are made particularly for the safety and security of women in India.

A. Sexual Harassment at Workplace

The Sexual Harassment at Workplace (Prevention, Prohibition and Redressal) Act, 2013 was enacted to guarantee the safety for women at workplaces and providing the environment that respects the dignity of women and provide them the equal status and opportunities. It applies to all women irrespective of age or employment, etc., and acts as a safeguard against their physical as well as mental harassment. This act boosts the women participation and decision-making power. For the effective implementation, there is an online complaint management system titled Sexual Harassment electronic-Box (SHe-Box) for making complaints related to harassment at workplaces.

B. Domestic Violence

With regards to the domestic violence, the key legislation is the Protection of Women from Domestic Violence Act (PWDVA), 2005. It envisages checking violence and providing immediate relief to the victims and letting women to breathe an open air at home. Protection officers in large numbers have been deployed to help women.

C. Dowry Prohibition

Another prevailing evil of dowry, which is deep rooted in the society, is a big threat for women empowerment. In this regard, the Dowry Prohibition Act was enacted in 1961. The Act implements checks on giving, taking or abetting of dowry. For the proper execution of the Act, the Dowry Prohibition Officers have been appointed.

D. Child Marriage

In 2006, The Prohibition of Child Marriage Act was implemented to restrict child marriages. It is a well-known subject of the National Plan of Action for Children, 2016. The concerned ministry makes advertisements through different media and educates people about the evils and consequence of child marriage. International Women Day and the National Girl Child Day are used to create awareness on issues related to women.

Constitutional Provisions for Empowering Women in India

- Article (14) - Equality before law for every person (Article-14).
- Article 15(I) - Prohibition of discrimination on grounds of religion, race, caste, sex or place of birth.
- (Article 16) - Equality of opportunity for all citizens relating to employment or appointment to any office under the state.
- (Article 39(a) - State policy to be directed to securing for men and women equally the right to an adequate means of livelihood.
- (Article 39(d) - Equal pay for equal work for both men and women.
- (Article 42) - Provisions to be made by the state for securing just and humane conditions of work and maternity relief.
- (Article 51A(e)) - Promotion of harmony by every citizen of India and renouncement of such practices which are derogatory to the dignity of women.
- (Articles 343(d) and 343 (T)) - Reservation of not less than one-third of total seats for women in direct election to local bodies, viz panchayats and municipalities.

Welfare Schemes for Women

A. Pradhan Mantri Matru Vandana Yojana (PMMVY)
The Scheme ensures to provide money in the form of cash to the pregnant (first child) and lactating mothers in three installments up to the amount of INR 5,000 in their accounts.

B. Mahila Shakti Kendra (MSK) Scheme
Mahila Shakti Kendra Scheme was approved in November, 2017 to uplift the women from rural areas in particular through community participation. It acts as an interface for women to approach governments for availing their entitlements and also strengthening them by imparting training and capacity building.

C. One Stop Centre
One Stop Centres (OSCs) have been set up for women facing violent crimes in the country which are named as Sakhi Centres. This scheme is working since 2015 to provide every needed service to women ranging from police, medical, legal, psychological support and temporary shelter to women affected by violence. Funding of

the scheme is made through Nirbhaya Fund. There is also a helpline for reporting the grievances.

D. Mahila Police Volunteers

This scheme is funded by Nirbhaya Fund as a centrally sponsored scheme with the aim to create and empower Mahila Police Volunteers (MPV). These volunteers act as a link between the police and community. They help women in solving their matters like domestic violence, child marriage, dowry harassment, etc.

E. Swadhar Greh

This scheme deals with the rehabilitation of women who meet unforeseen phase of life. It supports them to bring normality in their lives. Through this scheme, women are provided with shelter, food, clothing and medicines. Economic and social support is also extended to the victims which include widows, destitute women and aged women.

Conclusion

There is a changing scenario all over the world in the present era. Mindset towards women has been changing among the societies. Nowadays, laws and regulations are framed particularly to maintain the women dignity and to safeguard their rights as well. The issue of women empowerment has become the most vital concern of the 21st century globally. The governments of the world are not able to achieve this goal on their own, thus, the communities must come forward to join hands with the respective governments. There is a need to develop a conducive and favorable environment for women where then can breathe air of freedom and can enjoy respect, dignity and self-esteem. There shall be no gender based discrimination and women shall enjoy opportunities of self-decision making and participation in social, political and economic life of the country with a sense of equality.

India is experiencing a dynamic change over the period of time. There is a modification in the thoughts and outlook of the societies towards women. Slowly and steadily, there is an increase in the participation of women in making household decisions, and spousal violence has decreased with the spreading of more literacy and education. Women are also getting asset ownership rights and there is a considerable fall in the forced employment of women. As per NFHS-4, there is an increased percentage of women who earn more than their spouses, thus, signifying the capability of women to work at par with men. As compared to NFHS-3, an increased proportion of women are observed in NFHS-4 to go outside homes and are more exposed to media such as newspapers and television, thus, changing the obsolete mindset of the societies. More schooling and education has also led to all time high financial inclusion among women. There is an increase in the number of women who operate their bank accounts and make use of online money services, thus, taking advantages from microcredit programmes too.

With respect to the WPS Index, India is at the 5th position among the neighboring countries and has also excelled in three indicators of employment, mobile use and parliamentary representation.

It is said that a single woman nurtures a family. When a woman moves forward "the family moves, the village moves and the nation moves". It is very much indispensable that their thought and vision guide the development of a good family, good society and finally a good nation. Thus, women should be inducted in the mainstream of development. It can be effective and fruitful only when they own income and property so that they may become self-dependent and set up their identity in the society.

Women empowerment is a worldwide concept and needs to be addressed effectively and efficiently. Since the beginning, women have been facing gender based restrictions. Men have also supported and fought in favour of women over time. Until and unless women are given the same opportunities enjoyed by men, entire societies will perform below their potential. There would be inefficiency and less productivity. The biggest need of the hour is to bring change in the social attitude towards women in particular.

References

Rajeshwari, M. S. (2015). A Study on Issues and Challenges of Women Empowerment in India. *IOSR Journal of Business and Management (IOSR-JBM)*, 17(4), 13-19.

Rani, K., & Mercy, Sr. (2019). Women empowerment- a tool of national development. *Journal of Emerging Technologies and Innovative Research,* 6(3).

International Institute for Population Sciences (IIPS) and Macro International. (2007). *National Family Health Survey (NFHS-3), 2005–06:* India: Volume I. http://www.iipsindia.org or http://www.mohfw.nic.in

International Institute for Population Sciences (IIPS) and ICF. (2017). *National Family Health Survey (NFHS-4), 2015-16: India.* Mumbai: IIPS.

Government of India (2020). Annual Report 2019-20. Ministry of Women and Child Development. wcd.nic.in

Upadhyay,R. Women empowerment in India-an analytical overview. *The Asia Foundation.* asiafoundation.org. https://asiafoundation.org/resources/.../**womensempowermentindia**briefs.pdf.

Georgetown Institute for Women, Peace and Security and Peace Research Institute Oslo. (2019). *Women, Peace and Security Index 2019/20: Tracking sustainable peace through inclusion, justice, and security for women.* Washington, DC: GIWPS and PRIO.

12

Evolution of Women in Policing Around the World

Emil Jaison

Abstract

Women policing is not a newly developed role in our society. It can be dated all the way back to the mid-1800s. It formed its roots from the women's rights movement in America. Currently women police officers exist all around the world. They have equal footing in law enforcement as male officers. However, often, their duties and functions at work differ from their male colleagues. Such instances represent the gender imbalance within the system of law enforcement. Many societies around the world value the police officer post as a 'masculine' role. Culturally and traditionally in many parts of the world, women are considered weak, merely because of this reason they are regarded to be physically unfit to take on such roles. Despite these issues, women police have proved over the years that their presence as law enforcement officers is imperative for the secure handling of vulnerable women and children. This chapter discusses the evolution of women police on national and international levels and the influence various regional cultures and stereotypes when it comes to these female officers taking on such 'masculine' roles in the society.

Introduction

History is an important component in understanding the evolution of women in policing. History plays a major responsibility in comprehending the growth of a women police officer's position in our society. Women's role as a police officer has evolved over the years. Women police do not serve the same functions as the first police matron, or the same functions of the first female police officer. Their functions and duties have progressed throughout time. The purpose of a female police officer's role depends entirely upon the society and how they value women. Countries that follow liberal point of views toward the occupation of women are open towards women carrying on new roles in the society. On the other hand, countries that follow a strict regimen have predetermined notions as to what women ought to do in the society.

History of Women Policing

In the United States, the initiation towards employing female police officers arose in the 1880's. Such a movement was broadened with the help of several organizations such as Federation of Women's Clubs, the National League of Women Voters, the National Women's Christian Temperance Union, and various other local bodies. The aim of these national and local agencies was to arrange female figures, equivalent to police, who were efficient in handling cases related to women and girls. Such appointments were made to provide security to those held in police custodies, sent to prison, detention homes, mental asylums, and other public institutions.

These appointments were said to have been made as early as mid-1800's. In 1845, the American Female Society presided the appointments of female police matrons in the New York City Prison. In the 1870's, the Women's Christian Temperance was active in Portland, Maine, where the top members of the organization studied the livelihood of the female prisoners in the nearby prisons and simultaneously visited courts. They employed a female to visit prisons and later her role was raised to a 'police matron'.

Before the advent of woman police, primary appointments of female police were referred to as "police matrons". These matrons embarked the journey for the future of women policing in the United State of America. These earlier appointments were pivotal in history because they helped the society acknowledge that handling of women in law enforcement must come under the ambit of women. In the outset, police matrons were appointed for the secure handling of females in prison, assist male officers in cases involving women and children and attend court proceedings. The responsibilities and duties of police matrons and policewomen, who was later appointment, expanded over the years.

The first appointments of police matrons received positive feedback. Later such appointments were made throughout major cities and towns of United States. After the inception of the post of police matrons, laws were passed in the states of New York and Massachusetts addressing such appointments in 1888. The police matron post did not give women an equal standing to that of a male police officer, it was merely a safekeeping job. Women who held such posts purely went by the tag name 'worker' or 'operatives'. In 1909, a group of women from North Dakota urged the City Council to setup posts for policewomen in the City and, accordingly, an ordinance was passed in 1910, which gave the police matron posts identical powers to that of a police women.

It was Alice Stebbins Wells, from Los Angeles who became the first policewoman in America and in the world. Mrs. Wells who was a social worker, submitted a petition with signatures of 100 dominant figures to the City Mayor in seek of an appointment as a policewoman. Her petition was granted in 1910, making her the first policewoman. Her duties further extended to supervision, law enforcement in public places, and maintenance of information regarding women and children.

Many women groups came in support of Mrs. Wells for her appointment. In return, they demanded for lectures to empower the rest of the females in the community. These lectures helped the movement for women policing reach international level. Apart from conducting lectures in 73 cities in the US, Mrs. Wells was also invited to Canada to speak in front of a large audience in 1912. These lectures have influenced Canada in appointing its first female police matron later in the year.

Many organizations like Committee on Preventive Work for Women and Girls, the sections on Women and Girls of the Law Enforcement Division, the Women's Christian Temperance and others actively contributed towards educating the society and encouraging women to step forward to take such jobs considered to be virile by the society. This movement also helped in disclosing to the community that women are efficient in the field of law enforcement. Similarly, the society also came to realize that police officers are ideally social workers, who are working towards welfare and safety of the society by maintaining public order and enforcing law. They are at the lower strata when it comes to the hierarchy of civil servants. And yet they are the most important figures of the society because every case begins with a police complaint. This makes the police department the foundation and solution to many problems before letting them get intertwined in the judicial process. The female officers perfected the community by paying attention to small details that need straightening. Their initial roles were minor, and they dealt with vulnerable females in the society. They made good use of their role and proved to the society and authorities their capabilities to take on much serious roles within the system.

Appointments of policewomen were spreading from city to city in the late 1920s. After World War I, these appointments spread like a wildfire all around the country. It was a great vision to see women getting involved in law enforcement. However, none of this would have been made possible if not for women empowerment in the society. There are factors that lead to the success of the movement of women policing such as the expansion of freedom of women both at social and economic levels, their collective involvement in public affairs and involvement in political matters.

By 1915, the role of women in the police department extended to various other posts. Each department started appointing women for positions such as supervisor, superintendent, senior policewomen, and inspector posts. This opened new opportunities for women and increased their involvement in the community.

Division of Department into Units

Once the police departments started employing policewomen, the sudden increase in the number of women in the office started to have an impact on the organization of the departments. Communities started experimenting different methods for setting up the departments. They went about it in two ways, and they are as follows:

- Major cities featured more appointments due to the large number of applicants and this led to the creation of a women's division headed by Women officers in the police department.
- In smaller cities women were positioned in the already existing division which were headed by male officers.

Placing women under the supervision of male officers only limited their powers. On the other hand, big cities gave women the privilege of setting up women's division also referred to as women's bureau along with a female police officer as the director who enjoyed the same ranking as that of a male officer. Working in an empowering environment surrounded by strong and qualified women encouraged these women to be risk takers and be independent. Such a work environment provided women the liberty to develop and manage preventive programmes for women, children, and adolescents. It also helped in recruiting highly skilled women for the posts and establish training programmes specially for preparing women for such roles.

Having a separate women's division in the police department was a huge success. This new system received praises from the society and the leaders of the movement also urged the importance of such divisions within the department as it would concentrate the works of policewomen into one bureau. If these women were to scatter within the department, then their significance was bound to be lost. Majority of the successful crime deterrence work in the country during that time frame were conducted by women divisions. Therefore, it was important to set up more bureaus in the country. In 1922, the police chiefs passed a resolution in their annual meet which led to the formation of such women divisions in every police department. Despite this success, the smaller cities were gradual in establishing such divisions or bureaus within their departments.

The International Association of Policewomen (IAWP)

This association began with the labours of Alice Stebbins Wells, and she utilised her platform by taking the movement for women policing to reach international height. Her lectures inspired and influenced many young women. It started with the establishment of National Association of Policewomen on May 17th, 1915. Alice became the first president of this association. Prior to forming this association, Wells had acquired the consent of the International Association of Chiefs of Police and their support helped in drafting the constitution of the association.

The international association uplifted many women across the globe. Central office was in Washington D.C. The association over the course of time received calls from foreign countries to support the females of their society and empower their interest in women policing. An example was when Lady Nancy Astor from England called Alice to come and deliver a lecture to the women of England.

The association initially consisted of 320 members, mostly from North America and handful foreign members. Currently, the association is home to members from 73 countries and holds annual training conferences each year. Each year IAWP also provides scholarships to a remarkable woman officer to attend the annual training conference and all costs are borne by IAWP. The aim of this scholarship is to increase the role of women police across the globe and boost the membership of IAWP with more international participation. During these annual training conferences, selected women officers are given awards for their outstanding performance in the field of law enforcement. The women officers are recognized with awards for the following categories:

a) Officer of the year
b) Civilian of the year
c) Bravery
d) Leadership
e) Community service
f) Excellence in performance
g) Mentoring and coaching
h) Award in support of the UN "he for she" campaign
i) Prevention and detection of violence against women

International Perspective on Women Policing

The country to first introduce women policing is the United States, through the initiatives spread to the neighbouring countries and other places. In this journey, the English-speaking countries had begun the operation of recruiting women police in the early 1900s. Among these countries, United States commenced the movement by establishing the 'police matron' position in 1845. In the long run, this movement has influenced many other countries across the globe.

Canada: The first Canadian woman police officer is considered unofficially as Rose Fortune, an African American women, in the early 1800's, due to her remarkable contributions to the society. However, the post for women matron was instituted in 1912. This was followed by the lectures conducted by Alice Stebbins Wells in Canada the same year. Police matron's position was created to assist male officers in their works. It was in the year 1974 that a group of thirty-two women enrolled as women police officers. Ever since, the role of women police has broadened. Recently in 2018, Brenda Lucki has been appointed as the first female RCMP commissioner in Canada.

UK: The women were firstly appointed in the Metropolitan Police Department in 1919. They were police constables, whose job was to supervise public places. In 1919, the commissioner of police was Nevil Macready, who found women incompetent to do such 'male' roles in the society. However, in 1920, a committee was formed to recommend to the government regarding the extension of duties and functions of women police officers. This committee was chaired by Major Lawrence Baird, and the recommendations of this committee had a positive impact on the future role of women. In the later years, women's role as a police officer widened. They began working more closely towards women and children and later expanded to higher position in law enforcement.

Australia: Australia became an independent nation in 1901. The system of police was already established in the country by the Britishers before departing. Women were first appointed in the police services in 1915. Over the course of time, such appointments started to increase across the nation. The initial roles of women police were extremely subordinate and revolved around women and children. Often women police officers felt discriminated and marginalised in their workspace. After World War II, several women groups urged the government to reform the roles of these female officers. This proposal brought out change in the role of women police.

Brazil: In 1985, Brazil commenced its first All Women Police Unit (AWPU), and it comprised of only female staffs. These stations deal with cases in relation to offences against women and children. Apart from this, they are not assigned any traditional duties of police. This led to an issue of discrimination because any case that revolved around women and children were passed on to these units. Such issues were not given importance as compared other issues and they were not considered to be actual police work.

India: In India, the first female police officer was appointed in 1933 in Kerala. During the early days, women police dealt with cases involving only females and children. Eventually, their roles began advancing conventionally after enacting new labour laws in the country. In 1972, the first female officer was appointed as an IPS officer. There are All Women Police Units set up in various parts in India. These AWPUs are run solely by female staff. The women in India also serve at higher positions in mixed units as well, enjoying the same powers as men. However, women officers sometimes face discrimination from their male colleagues.

Middle East: In the Arab countries, women police officers were appointed in the 1970's. Oman and Bahrain were the first to start the movement in the Middle East. Subsequently, UAE and Qatar also joined the list in the 1980's and 1990's. Kuwait appointed the first female police officers in 2011. These regions have special units made up of women officers. They deal with matters in relation to women and children. These units are specialised to handle crimes against housemaids or foreign domestic workers.

South Africa: In South Africa, the women officers were appointed in the 1990s. In 1997, South Africa started the initiative for gender balance within the units. In 2017, 27.5% of the police service consisted of women. Along with the increased involvement, top official positions were also filled by women. They have been encouraged to apply for promotions. Trainings are also set up for educating these officers on the country's sexual harassment policy and for building leaderships skills. However, the crime rate against women is still high even after recruiting high number of women in the police.

Finland: Female police officers were appointed to look after matters regarding women and children. Later, several NGO advocated to the government to initiate training programmes for women police officers. Things were not in the favour of these women police officers till World War II. After the war, state police school training was initiated. Since 1970s, equal footing in police services were given to both males and females. Most of the women police officers in the country are highly educated and qualified. However, some discrimination still exists in the field of promotions.

Poland: Women started their career in the police service in 1925. In the early days, women served subordinate roles in the police service. Eventually, after many reforms, the women officer's role developed equally as that of male officers. Women officers are generally highly educated. However, some discrimination still exists.

Singapore: A group of ten women were given police constable roles initially. Police constables have a subordinate role in the police department, and they are assigned to do clerical work. Out of these ten women, Mary Voon was assigned in 1949 to be the first female police inspector. In 1970s, women were recruited as traffic police. This appointment broke a lot of conventions and treated women at par with men. Since 1980s, female officers have been given equal tasks as men. Women also started serving high positions in the police.

Each country has its own rational for launching this movement in the nation. In USA, the reason for introducing the post of police matron was for the secure handling of women in prisons, and the duties and responsibilities augmented over the course of time. Similarly, in many Asian countries like Singapore, Japan, Indonesia, etc., women police were appointed to protect women from the social and economic conditions prevailing at the time of appointment. In some other countries, like Germany, women police were assigned to oversee and enforce laws pertaining to prostitution. Most of the Middle Eastern countries have delegated women police at check posts and security check-ins at public places for safe conduct and supervision of females.

United Nations Peacekeepers

United Nations peacekeepers consists of police, civilians and military. The police peacekeepers ensure that female participation in law enforcement is achieved. Women police are prototypes of gender equality, and their services help inspire many young women to enter this field of public service. Their role helps the UN in dismantling sexual exploitation and abuse against women and children prevalent in our society.

The UN peacekeeping started in 1945, and it consisted of all men. It was formed to maintain peace and security in the world. Till 1992, only 1% of the force comprised of women, and most of the women served in the medical units as doctors and nurses. The low deployment was due to the absence of any UN policy for the induction of women into UN peacekeeping. The UN civilian police forces deeply lacked the involvement of women, which led them to borrow female officers from the military force. Then, as a solution to this predicament, in 1994, the UN requested its member nations to sanction women officers to join the UN peacekeeping. USA, France and Australia were the first countries to respond to UN's request. Women police from these countries were sent to join various UN missions. Even then, UN found difficulty in gathering representation of women from all its member states because some countries were displeased to have their women participate in such missions.

In 2009, after realizing the low number of women police serving in the UN, the UN took efforts and increased these numbers by recruiting more women to work for UN as police peacekeepers. The initiative was called 'Global Effort' and it was for maintaining gender balance among UN peacekeepers. For this UN worked closely with the signatory states and national police services around the world. It increased the number from 900 women officers to 1,300 in 2016. For the 'Global Effort', the member nations were requested to do the following by the United Nations:

- Create a national policy to ensure that the percentage of women police is in parity with the country's national police gender ratio.
- Female candidates shall be encouraged to take part in the international peacekeeping recruitment procedures.
- Incentives to be provided to officers who operated in the UN peacekeeping missions.

Trainings were conducted by the United Nations Police Division for enlisting eligible candidates as United Nations Police Officer. These trainings helped the women in preparing for the recruitment tests that they needed to pass to be selected for the United Nations Police Division.

The partaking of women in the UN peacekeeping missions has been an eyeopener for the UN in terms of understanding gender and human rights issues involving females and children. It has also been observed that female victims are receptive towards female officers than male officers. For instance, in the UN mission in Ghana, the females present at the refugee camps were willing to converse with the women police about incidents of sexual exploitation and abuse involving them. This reveals that the participation of females in the police forces is essential for providing support and strengthening the laws in relation to female victims and children.

Conclusion

The role of women in policing has helped women break the conventional role the society had tattooed on women. The duties and functions of a women officer has also evolved over the course of the years. Countries like United States and England have long history regarding women in policing. The role of women police officers began as protective figures to look after women, adolescents, and children in the society. Over the course of time, their duties and responsibilities magnified, and they came in parity with the male officers. Many traditional and developing countries like Brazil, India, Taiwan, Bahrain, and UAE have female police officers present in their societies, but their role as a police officer is gender specific. Due to this, the women police in these countries work in an All Women Police Units (AWPU). Thus, there is a need for achieving more equality in the role of women police in many countries. Women divisions, at the same time, have made women officers feel more encouraged and liberated in their workspace. In these divisions, women are exposed to higher positions in the field of law enforcement. They do not have to worry about anyone questioning their credibility or face sexual harassment at workplace. This means than the inclusion of women in police service must be increased to eliminate the crime rate, and such increase can lead to safe workspaces for women in police. However, increasing the number of women in police is not the only measure to be taken to decrease the crime rate in a country. Along with employing more women police officers, the initiatives should be developed to reduce the crimes against women and children.

References

Canada, I. A. (2020, September 26th). *Canadian History of Women in Policing.* Retrieved from International Association of Women Police Canada: http://iawp.cpsevents.ca/2018/05/31/canadian-history-of-women-in-policing/

Cells, O. P. (2020, September 28th). *History of Women in the Police Force.* Retrieved from Old Police Museum Cells: https://www.oldpolicecellsmuseum.org.uk/content/history/women_police_officers/history_of_women_in_the_police_force

Denney, L. (2019). *Gender and Seecurity Toolkit: Policing and Gender.* Genev: Geneva Center for Security Sector Governance.

Garcia, C. R.-H. (2019). *Women Policing Across the Globe.* London: Rowman and Littlefield.

Higgins, L. (1951). Historical Background of Policewomen's Service. *Journal of Criminal Law and Criminology*, 13.

United Nations (1995). *Women 2000.* New York: Division for the Advancement of Women.

Ng, R. (2020, September 28th). *Evolution of Women in Policing.* Retrieved from Singapore Police Force: https://www.police.gov.sg/media-room/features/the-evolution-of-women-in-policing

IAP (2020, September 25th). *Annual Recognition Programme.* Retrieved from International Association of Women Police : http://www.iawp.org/annual-recognition

UN Police (2020, September 29th). *Recruiting more Police Women .* Retrieved from United Nations Police : https://police.un.org/en/recruiting-more-police-women

UN Police (2020, September 29th). *UN Police Gender Initiatives.* Retrieved from United Nations Police : https://police.un.org/en/un-police-gender-initiatives

Rao, B. (2020, September 28th). *Women in the Police Force – Numbers & Beyond.* Retrieved from Factly: https://factly.in/women-in-the-police-force-numbers-beyond/

Williams, K. (2020, September 29th). *Breaking the Brass Ceiling: Policewomen Around the World.* Retrieved from Inclusive Security: https://www.inclusivesecurity.org/2014/05/13/policewomen-around-world/

Woodeson, A. (1993). The first women police: a force for equality or infringement? *Women's History Review* , 17.

13

Different Strategies to Protect Girls from Early Marriage Since the Era of Vidyasagar to Covid-19 Period

Sujit Samanta

Abstract

The ongoing Covid-19 crisis has changed social and economic scenario of whole world. Unemployment, economic hardships and livelihood challenges have made an impact on the poorest women and girls. Many families have chosen to marry their girls off due to the destruction of livelihood. Two hundred years ago, Vidyasagar started the movement to stop the child marriage, today we are in a state to restart this movement to save our girl child. The objectives of the study are 1) to study the concept of child marriage as perceived in the era of Vidyasagar, 2) to find out impact of Covid-19 on child marriages in today's times and 3) to find out the strategies to prevent child marriage in post Covid-19 period. First child marriage Act was came into force in 1891 after the long social reforms movement by Vidyasagar. Vidyasagar pointed out the bad effects of child marriage through this writings and started girls' education in colonial Bengal. However, the child marriage tradition is still running in many marginal families our society. It has been observed to increase in the Covid-19 period owing to the breakdown of economic condition during lockdown. To make an Atmanirbhar Bharat, we should protect our girls from early marriage through community awareness in the post Covid-19 period.

Introduction

"As Covid-19 forces school closures in 185 countries, Plan International and UNESCO warn of the potential for increased drop-out rates which will disproportionately affect adolescent girls, thus, further entrenching the gender gaps in education and leading to an increased risk of sexual exploitation, early pregnancy and early marriage."- Stefania Giannini, UNESCO Assistant Director General (Education) and Anne Birgitte Albrectsen, Chief executive Officer, Plan International (UNESCO, June, 2020).

The ongoing Covid-19 crisis has changed social and economic scenario in the whole world. Numerous people have already died due to the pandemic. During this period, the systems and institutions for provision of essential service to females have been badly affected. These include police, health, legal aid, justice, counselling centres, shelters, etc. Unemployment, economic hardships and livelihood challenges have impacted the poorest women and girls the most. As per a UNESCO report, 111 million girls are devoid of education. Many families choose to marry their girls off due to the livelihood issues. Two hundred years ago Vidyasagar started a movement to stop child marriage, and there is a need to restart this movement today. Union Finance Minister Nirmala Sitharaman during her budget session speech on 29th Feb 2020 also announced to frame a task force to consider raising the age for marriage.

Child marriage is a global threat. As per a **World Bank** report, "Child marriage is also a critical challenge. Child brides are much more likely to drop out of school and complete fewer years of education than their peers who marry later. This affects the education and health of their children as well as their ability to earn a living." World Bank said "more than 41000 girls under the age of 18 marry every day, and putting an end to the practice would increase women's expected education attainment, and with it their potential earnings. According to estimates, ending child marriage could generate more than £500 billion in benefits annually each year."

As per a **UNICEF** report, at least 1.5 million girls under 18 get married in India, 1/3 of total global child marriages (the table below).

Year	Married before their 18th birthday (Indian women)
2005-2006	47%
2015-2016	27%

Thus, it is needed to achieve gender equality and empowerment of all women and girls, by eliminating the practices such as early and forced marriages. UNICEF and UNFPA have taken joint initiatives to accelerate action to end child marriage.

Indian Human Development Survey 2004 -05 remarked that 95% of Indian women are married by age of 25.

Year	Mean Age of Marriage of women
1961	16.1
1991	19.3
1998-99	19.7

Source: Survey DLHS 2007-2008

Literature Review

"Polygamy, child marriage, ascetic widowhood and prostitution as well as denial of education to women are now widely believed to be the major issues affecting the lives of women in nineteenth-century Bengal." **(Anisuzzaman 2000. Chakrabarti 1998 & Murshid 1984). Zafar (2014)** remarked that "during his lifetime, Vidyasagar campaigned against polygamy, child marriage and prostitution. He also argued strongly in favour of women's education." **Mitra, Chandra and Subal** remarked "Vidyasagar's maturely gentle and compassionate heart was moved at the sight of the tender young widows suffering rigorous hardships, and he was firmly resolved to devote his life to the cause of the remarriage of Hindu widows." As per **Adhakari (1980),** Vidyasagar perceived that women in India were the downtrodden and tormented section of society. His compassionate heart melted at the pitiable condition of their lives, and he was determined to fight for the right of women. It was a great challenged for him, and he accepted the challenge. **Shrivavastava, Shrivastava and Ramasamy (2016)** pointed that "there is an extensive need to discourage any practices prevalent in the society which favor discrimination against the girls or reduces the opportunities for girls and young women. We have to involve more numbers of people in the battle against child marriage."

Objectives of Study

1) to study the concepts child marriage as perceived in the era of Vidyasagar
2) to find out impact of Covid-19 on child marriages in today's times
3) to find out the strategies to prevent child marriage in post Covid-19 period

Population and sample: The population of the study is the girls who have been married below the age of eighteen. The sample has nee collected from ten families of two districts of West Bengal state.

Data: Primary data was collected from ten families where child marriage has happened in two district of West Bengal. The secondary data has been obtained collected from writings of Vidyasagar, journals and online sources.

Methodology: This study is an analytical survey. A case study was conducted with ten families where girls had been married below 18 years age. A non-formal interview was taken with their guardians.

Analysis and Findings

The concept of child marriage as perceived in the era of Vidyasagar: Hindu marriage may be solemnized between any two Hindus if they fulfill all the condition as laid down in the Hindu Marriage Act. From the patriarchal society of Rig Vedic Hindus, marriage was considered as a sacramental union. The rites and ceremonies include the Saptpadi (the taking of seven steps by the bridegroom and the bride jointly before the sacred fire), and the marriage becomes complete and binding when the seventh step is taken. The social reform movements characteristic of the first half of the 19th century addressed predominantly the "women question." Through his writing, Vidyasagar motivated the urban middle classes for widow remarriage and against child marriage and polygamy. Vidyasagar wrote:

- Child marriage adversely affects the health of the bride, and it hinders their education.
- The child bride faces the health related problem.
- Danger of early widowhood.
- Both husband and wife are not mature at the tender age.

It was perhaps the most difficult task in the 19th century in Bengal. Number of widows had increased due to child marriage and polygamy. He did not stop after the Widow Remarriage Act was passed in 1856. First widow remarriage took place on 7th December 1856 under his supervision. The bride was 10 year old Smt. Kalimati. She had becomes a widow at the age of 6.

To uplift the status of female Vidyasagar understood the necessity for the reformation of Bengali Marriage Act. Age Consent Act 1891 was passed after the long movement by Vidyasagar and others.

Vidyasagar also wanted to reform Hindu marriage customs through the eye of humanism. Gopal Haldar remarked that the strategies of social reforms adopted by Vidyasagar represented scientific humanism.

Impact of Covid-19 on child marriages: Covid-19 pandemic has affected the world economy. Specifically, it has enhanced the economic suffering, vulnerability and gender disparities in education and social sector. Covid-19 has also led to a digital divide in rural India. One group of students have access to the internet and technology (mobile/television and personal computer), whereas the other is deprived of these. The girl students are observed to be more severely impacted by this situation. Many families have no capacity to provide food to their children during pandemic. The migrant labourers have been forced to return to their homes. As many people have lost the economic means, thus, child labour, early marriage, child abuse and human trafficking will be increased in post Covid19 period, as per report of National Commission of Women.

Prevention strategies of child marriage in post Covid-19 period: The reasons behind the child marriage are identified as poverty, superstition, geographical location, lack of communication, natural disasters, lack of education, etc. Role of NGOs, child helplines and police should be prompted on child marriage. There are many government scheme like Bati Bacho Bati Parao and Kanayashree, which have proven to be very effective in reducing the child marriages. However, in the post Covid-19 situation, there will be a tendency to initiate the child marriage due to the economic breakdown of the society. Girls children of migrant labourers and families of socially disadvantaged groups are specifically at risk.

Causes of Child Marriage in Vidyasagar and Post Covid-19 Periods

No.	Cause of child marriage in the era of Vidyasagar	Cause of child marriage in post Covid-19 period
1.	Social superstition	Patriarchal society, gender stereotype concepts
2.	Castesiam, dowry, poverty, and no reforms movements.	Dowry, poverty, etc. However, Child Marriage Act has came in force.
3.	No schooling facilities, only	Schooling facility and government

	higher caste girls used to go to school	incentives are available, however, the guardians are not motivated to educate their girls
4.	Colonial period, guardians did not encourage their girls to study	Less political willingness to stop child marriage
5.	Education was not free	Education is free, but tuition is needed
6.	Agriculture based village economy	MGNREGS and MSME schemes are available to empower village economy, but marginal families do not get the benefit.

A case study has been carried out by selecting ten families from two districts of West Bengal where child marriage has taken place. A non-formal interview was conducted with the guardians.

No.	Name of the district (West Bengal)	Block	Age of marriage	No. of families	No of guardians participated in the Interview
1.	Purulia	Jalda	Below 18 years	5	5
2.	North 24 Parganas	Kakdip	Below 18 years	5	5

The following table presents the outcome of the interviews:

	Status of girls and reason of child marriage
1.	All families are from economically weaker section of the society.
2.	Seven girls are studying in the schools, and three are out of school.
3.	School going girls are not interested in studying as the tuition fees is not provided by the families.
4.	The fathers of some girls are migrant labourers. The guardians feel unsafe leaving the girls alone, so they arrange for their marriage. Some have lost their work due to the pandemic, thus, enhancing the economic hardship.
5.	The guardians mentioned that the suitable match from a boy's families with no dowry demand makes them accept the child marriage.
6.	Amfan cyclone led to a widespread destruction, thus, making them more insecure.

Conclusion

Covid-19 has reignited the menace of child marriage. It is of utmost importance to stay vigilant and empower the women of the country so as to achieve a healthy development of everyone in the society, which, in turn, benefits the communities, regions and countries.

References

Adhikari, K. S. (1980) *Vidyasagar and the Regeneration of Bengal*, Subarnarekha, Calcutta.

Bhola, Venkateswarm, and Koul. *Corona Epidemic in Indian Context: Predictive   Mathematical   Modelling*, https://doi.org/10.1101/2020.04.03.200117175.

Gender and COVID 19 (Coronavirus), World Bank Group. Retrieved on July 12, 2020 from https://www.worldbank.org

Ghose, J., Dubey, Chatterjee and S. Dubey (2020) Impact of COVID-19 on children: special focus on the psychological aspect. *Minerva Pediatrica*, http://www.minervamedica.it

Impact of COVID-19 on violence against women and girls and service provision. Retrieved on July 12, 2020 from https://www.unwomen.org 2020/04

Mitra, C. S. (1902) *Iswar Chandra Vidyasagar: A story of his life and work*, Ashish Publication, New Delhi.

Zafar, M. (2014) Social Reform in Colonial Bengal: Revisiting Vidyasagar, Philosophy and Progress, Vols, LV-LVI, p. 111.

Government of India (2000) *The Right of children to Free and Compulsory Education for Children*, New Delhi, GOI.

Government of India (1883-84) Indian Education Commission, Report and Appendices, Calcutta.

Halder, G. (1972) *Vidyasagar: A Reassessment*, West Bengal Public Library Network, p. 44.

Mitra, Indra (September 2001) *Karunasagar Vidyasagar*, Ananda Publishers, Calcutta.

NCERT (2005) The National Curriculum Framework (NCF, 2005), New Delhi, Govt. of India.

Roy, K. A. (2018) Ishwar Chandra Vidyasagar: The Champion Educator of Bengal. *The Research Journal of Social Sciences*, November 2018, Vol. 9, No. 11.

Shrivavastava S. R., Shrivastava, P. S. and Ramasamy, J. (2016) Ending Child Marriage: Battling for a Girls' Right to Choose. Primary Health Care (2016), Vol 6, Issue 1.

Sen, Asok (2016) *Iswar Chandra Vidyasagar and His Elusive Milestones*, Ashoka University, New Delhi.

14

Women Workers' Rights and Gender Equality: A Critical Analysis

Rima Ghosh
Santanu Panda

Abstract

In this article, a literature-based study has been carried out to explore the state of the women workers in our society. Women have been considered as the weaker section of the society for long. However, women have a vital role to play globally. It is extremely important to make the women workers aware about their legal rights The legal rights of the workers, especially women, are one of the most fundamental objectives of ILO. Equality and safety of women in all organised and unorganised working sectors is an important goal for achieving equitable justice. In earlier days, women were uneducated and not allowed to go out of the home. After independence, the women have gradually attained education and have also come forward to fight against the social evils. They have established an identity of their own in different areas of work. Since 1970's, the government has tried to bring them in the mainstream by implementing various schemes. For instance, PHN, ANM, GNM, ICDS, SHG, ASHA, ANM, etc., provide exclusively women oriented jobs in India. However, the work of many women workers is still not documented. This is due to the reason that a majority of women workforce is engaged in the unorganized sector. It is recommended that an appropriate reservation for women should be implemented in both education and employment.

Introduction

The rate of participation of the women workers in India is much lower than men. Among the women, the employment levels of urban women are lower than that of their rural counterparts. Further, the conditions of the women workers at the work place in India are inferior as compared to the Western countries. Moreover, there are no old age schemes. This clearly indicates the women suffering from unemployed and lack of financial support would be completely dependent on their spouses and family members, and their family sometimes considers them as a burden. Again, in some parts of the country, there are orthodox customs against women that a woman going out for work brings down the man's dignity and status in the society, as men are always considered superior than women. This kind of scenario mostly prevails in the rural India. It is like other side of the coin in the urban areas of India that women take active participation in the working sector. For instance, in the metropolitan cities, around 2/3rd of women work in IT industry, hotel industry and many other sectors of business.

The economy of India has been on the highflyer on the world stage in the recent years. In the year 2017, it has become one of the fastest growing country in terms of economy, with GDP growth above 7% p.a. However, since 2017, the participation of women work force has been somehow reduced in India. The World bank has also reported that India and other Asian countries have low women workforce.

The main reason for the decline of women workers in India are as follows:
o   The ratio of women in the occupational sectors is low.
o   Everything has become automatic, thus, less workforce.
o   As the wealth of the each household in the society is increasing, it leads the women to drop out.
o   Women do not get much support from their family members.

Status of Women Workers in India

It has been seen from the history that every society differentiates between the sexes. The people residing in the society always consider men as superior than women, and, therefore, the women jobs are largely in lower categories. However, in the modern period, the laws have granted equality in the status of men and women. However, there are difficulties in actually implementing these laws. In the cities, the women are coming up for their rights as implemented in the law owing to increase awareness.[1] Even women are sometimes

---

[1]Omen, T. K. and Venugopal C. N. "Sociology" Eastern Book Company, Lucknow, 1993, Page 360

considered as a handicapped during their pregnancy or maternity period by the society. *"The dependency period of a human infant is one of the longest and the women have to bear the brunt of it. These biologically anchored but culturally reinforced feminine roles gave birth to the argument that human bio grammar is geared to sexual division of labour in society."* From the history itself, in the early ages, the people were mostly dependent on hunting for their livelihood. Thus, men were politically strong and capable enough to protect their community. This was the reason that men those days were considered superior to women. This has become cultural tradition which is still on going in the modern day societies.

When the concept of gender equality comes in discussion in the society, the main motive is the equality in status between men and women in every sector. The Indian religious books have always mentioned womanhood as a gift of God as it brings new life in the world. Woman is considered as the creator of the universe. According to the scriptures, women should be treated with dignity, honour and respect in the society. However, the women are seen to be lagging behind in the society. Every human being has the fundamental right of equality and justice which are the prime motive of the human rights in the world. In globalized world, gender equality is valued. When men and women work together hand in hand, it can be envisaged to lead to a cherished society across the globe. There is requirement to spread awareness in the society and making the people understand about the importance of woman for the entire society.

Empowerment of Women Workers

The concept of women empowerment has become one of the most principal concepts and a topic of discussion in the world. This concept will help the women to receive the chance to express their views and to achieve the same status, respect and dignity as men in the society. If women are given same status in the society as men, they can also flourish in their respective fields. Moreover, if power and position are given to women, they can even perform better than their competitors. The empowerment of women is not only important for society, but also equally important at the homes. In this context, the self-help groups (SHGs) have played an important role in promoting the empowerment and development of women.

In the tribal of the states of Telangana, the women with the help of SHGs have achieved to bring in limelight on the issue of women empowerment. SHGs is an important organization mainly helping the tribal women. For instance, it provides chances for the tribal women of Telangana to engage themselves in several small cottage industries. Due to this, SHGs in India have created a movement for the development of women. The empowerment of women workers is vital in the modernized world as the country will only flourish if women are given equality in all respects. The empowerment of women workers is also vital for the socio-economic development of the society. Thus, the women should also come forward as a focal point for the development of the nation.

The rural woman are the centre of the rural development in terms of alleviation of rural poverty. Therefore, the government has initiated women self-help group programme as a participatory approach for rural development as well as eradication of rural poverty. However, the Ninth Plan notices that in spite of development measures and constitutional guarantees, the women have lagged behind in almost all sectors. Though the government has continued to allocate resources and formulated policies for the empowerment of women, it has become clear that political and social forces, that resist women's rights in the name of religious, cultural or ethnic traditions, have contributed to the process of marginalization and oppression of women. Poverty and unemployment are the major challenges of the under developed countries. In India, at the end of Ninth Five Year plan, 26% of the population was living below the poverty line in the rural area. The overall unemployment rate was 8.5%, and the rate of growth of women unemployment in the rural areas was 9.8%. Thus, the development of the rural sector and rural women is the main need of the Indian economy.

Self-Help Groups

Self-help group (SHGs) is a vital concept of women empowerment. It has great role in hastening country's economic development. SHGs have now evolved as a movement. A SHG is a village-based financial intermediary usually composed of 10-15 local women. All members have regular savings contributions over few months until there is enough capital in the group to begin lending. It has been realized in many parts of the world that an effective way to tackle poverty and to enable communities to improve the quality of life is through social mobilization of disadvantaged people, especially into SHGs. The SHGs also play an important role in elevating the economic status of their families. This has led to boosting the process of women's empowerment. In the recent years, empowerment has been recognized as the central issue in determining the status of women. As women become more potent source of development, empowering them is a prerequisite for overall development. The economic status of women is now accepted as an indicator of an economy's level of development. The empowerment seeks to meet women's strategic gender needs, through bottom up mobilization. It aims at increasing women's power in terms of their self-reliance and internal strength to make choices in life and to influence the direction of change.

Rights of Women Workers at Work Place

Law against sexual harassment: In 2013, the Sexual Harassment of Women at Workplace (Prevention, Prohibition, and Redressed) Act was enacted to help those facing the sexual harassment at work. Owing to this Act, every company must have a well-documented mechanism to address complaints about sexual advances and demands for sexual favours at work.

Law for maternity benefits
   o 26 weeks of paid maternity leave
   o One month of paid leave for any illness due to pregnancy or miscarriage
   o Medical bonus of INR 2,500 to Rs 3,500 if the employer provides pre-natal and post-natal care
   o Maternity benefit when the employee shows proof of delivery, to be paid 48 hours in advance
   o When the employee dies leaving no legal heir, a nominated beneficiary gets the maternity benefit.

Law for factory workers: Proper working conditions include ensuring health, safety, welfare, proper working hours, leave, and other benefits. Women workers must get 24 hours' notice if there is a change in their shift timings. If a factory hires more than 30 women workers, it has to have a crèche for children aged six years and below.

Law for equal pay: The Equal Remuneration Act and Article 39 of the Indian Constitution make it compulsory to pay an equal pay to the men and women. Employers must pay male and female employees equally for the same position. Also, employers cannot discriminate against women during the hiring process.

Law for protecting women during night shifts: The Shops and Establishment Act protects the women employees who work during the night shifts. The employers must apply for approvals if they need to work beyond prescribed limits. The approvals include conditions such as providing sufficient security and conveyance during night shifts.

Scenario of Gender Equality

Globally, women have fewer opportunities for economic participation than men, less access to basic and higher education, greater health and safety risks, and less political representation. Guaranteeing the rights of women and giving them opportunities to reach their full potential is critical not only for attaining gender equality, but also for meeting a wide range of international development goals. Empowered women and girls contribute to the health and productivity of their families, communities, and countries, creating a ripple effect that benefits everyone.

The gender equality agenda is based on the fundamental principles of democracy, social justice, human rights and human resource management. Gender equality entails reducing barriers based on sex differences and eliminating any form of discrimination based on gender classification, a process requiring definition of the current situation by means of both quantitative and qualitative data.

Women's satisfaction, 'self-actualisation' and self-confidence contribute to improve the quality of life for both sexes and for individuals. It is not possible to achieve these goals without strengthening and enlarging national institutional structures for gender equality. Options in this regard include a separate parliamentary committee on gender equality and even a government ministry, as well as an ombudsman. The establishment of an overall authority, for example, a governmental council for gender equality should be considered seriously.

Objective of the Study

The following objectives are applied to realise the situation of the women workers and their rights, namely
- o To know the role of women in the family and society.
- o To find the literature regarding the women participation in PRI (Panchayat Raj Institution).
- o Finally, the putting forward a few policy oriented measures to promote gender equality and protect women workers' rights in our society.

Methodology

The study conceptualizes the theoretical insights through the literature review. It is purely based on doctrinal study. The ideas and thoughts have been backed by eminent scholars of the contemporary generation.

Discussion

Participation of women in the Panchayat Raj Institution: The 73rd constitutional amendment on reservation for women was fiercely debated. Many politicians were skeptical whether women in villages would come forward to fill the stipulated 33% positions in village governance. Their doubts were, however, belied. Today, there are more women in panchayats than the stipulated 33%, and many states have raised women quota to 50 per cent. Bihar was the first state to do so, and 54% of elected representatives of PRI's in Bihar today are women. In Himachal Pradesh, there are over 57% women in the tree tire Panchayat Raj Institutions, 451 women have been elected from the unreserved seats in the state. Several other states including Uttarakhand, Tripura, MP, AP, Kerala, Maharashtra, and Rajasthan have reserved 50 percent seats for woman in panchayats. There is no doubt that reservation for women in panchayats opened the door for their empowerment at the grassroots level. As the Centre for Women's Development Studies in 1999 revealed, 95% of women surveyed felt that they would not have been elected had it not been for the reservation.

It has been observed from several examples and various literature studies that women have played a vital role in the society, e.g., campaigns against liquor consumption, child marriages and other evils in the society. They have not only worked for ensuring development of villages but have also organized self-help groups for their economic empowerment.[2,3]

Role of women in family: The health of the family significantly depends on women. A woman has a vital role in family planning, child health, child education, female education and girl child advocacy. A woman is a good policy-maker in a family for smooth running of the family. Thus, the women are the backbone of a family as well as a society.

Hirway (1985) studied the working of the Maternity Benefits Act in the state of Gujarat and concluded that less than 2.5% of women workers in the state were covered by the Act, about one-fifth of these (or 0.5%) actually received the benefits, and only a portion of these in turn received all the benefits laid down by law. In general, the employers considered women workers less reliable, less efficient, and more expensive, and so tried to avoid giving women long-term employment and denied them maternity benefits. At the same time, women's weak bargaining power in the labor market discouraged them from fighting for their rights. Implementation of the Act by the government was also quite inefficient. Hirway concludes that the Maternity Benefits Act does not really help to protect women's employment or look after the health of working mothers or their infants, therefore, failing in its prime responsibility to enable women to work and carry out family responsibilities.[3]

Violence against women: In our country, many instances of violence against women take place, e.g., child marriage, women trafficking, crime against adolescent girls, exploitation of the differently abled women, prostitution, etc.

Legal status of women in India: The Indian constitution has considered women as the legal citizens of our country. Therefore, women have been granted equal rights as men. However, many women

---

[2]Susmita Bera, 'Women and Panchayati Raj Systems' in the Kurukhetra, a journal of Ministry of rural Development, 2015.
[3]Hirway, Indira (1985), "Denial of Maternity Benefits to Women Workers in India - A Study of Factory Sector in Gujarat", Gandhi Labour Institute, Ahmedabad.

are malnourished and in poor health. Many Indian women are still illiterate. The women are required to take care of household works and handle the daily activities. This creates a major problem with nutrition, especially at the time of pregnancy or nursing. Very few women seek medical care for health related issues. This is also one of the main reasons of India's high maternal and infant mortality rates. Even right of education is provided by constitution of India, however, only about 39% of all women in India actually attend primary schools. So even though the education does not financially burden the family, the time the girl students spend at school is considered by the male dominated families as a wastage of time. However, the status of women in India has been subject to many changes over the span of recorded Indian history. Women in India are being provided with the legal security to secure their economic, social and cultural aspirations. The following legislation show the efforts made by Indian government in safeguarding the interests of women.

- Dowry Prohibition Act 1961;Maternity Benefit Act 1861,
- Births, Deaths & Marriages Registration Act 1886; Medical Termination of Pregnancy Act 1971,
- National Commission for Women Act 1990,
- Pre-natal Diagnostic Techniques (Regulation and Prevention of Misuse) Act 1999,
- Protection of Women from Domestic Violence Act 2005,
- Sexual Harassment of Women at Work Place (Prevention, Prohibition & Redressal) Act 2013,
- Hindu Widows Remarriage Act 1856; Muslim Women (protection of rights on divorce) Act 1986; Guardians and Wards Act 1890,
- Indian Penal Code 1860; Christian Marriages Act 1872, etc.

The education of women in India has played a significant role in improving their livings standards. A high women literacy rate improves the quality of life both at home and outside.

Status of women: The government of India took up the national plan of action for women in 1976. The government of India made yet another attempt to focus on the issues of women and development by putting a separate chapter on this subject in Sixth Plan. In this plan, the crucial issues affecting women in the field of health, education, employment and social welfare were focused on. In the

Seventh Plan, a chapter entitled "Socio-economic Programmes for Women" was added. In its review of the Sixth Plan, the only achievements the chapter could mention were the creation of a special cell in the employment ministry to look after the provisions of the Equal Remuneration Act applicable to the organised sector, catering to only 12.9 percent of the women workers. The 1976 plan of action had suggested setting up of standing advisory committee at the national level called the National Committee on Women which was supported to meet every year so that a report could be submitted to the Parliament annually. The central and state social welfare boards also implemented various welfare programmes for women. However, more needs to be still achieved to fulfill the goal of women empowerment.[4]

The government initiated various job-oriented strategies for the development of women. Health, education, employment and social justice are the key indicators of women development. Historically, the planning approach for women's development since 1st five-year plan has moved from concentration on the welfare approach to women's problems. For example, in Rajasthan, a variety of social, cultural and historical factors have conspired to give rise to a condition that may be described as extremely adverse to women. The legacy of a feudal structure is particularly manifest in the social isolation of women. The literacy rate for women in Rajasthan is only 11.4% as compared to the national figure of 24.82%. Further, the literacy rate of SC women is only 1.18%, whereas it is only 0.93 percent for the ST women according to 2011 census. The scenario for women vis-à-vis health and nutrition is particularly bleak. Anemia is a very high-risk factor in maternal mortality. Discrimination against the women by employers has also been commonly observed.[5] Overall, women play a vital role in the labour force, and their contribution to the national economy is beyond doubt. The women suffer from various forms of discrimination both in the organized and unorganized sectors, and the development of an equal society is the need of the hour.

---

[4]Sudhir Varma "Status of women in India, Policy Planning and the implementation machinery: some crucial issues" published in edited book entitled: *Administration for empowerment and welfare of women* by Abha Jain &SaliniShekharvat, 2007.

[5]Malavika Pawar, "Some strategies for women's development" published in edited book entitled: *Administration for empowerment and welfare of women* by Abha Jain &SaliniShekharvat, 2007.

Conclusion

The article concludes that the women are still the neglected part of the society. The paper has also highlighted the discrimination against the women in the work place in both organized or unorganized sectors. Violence against women and gender inequality are observed to occur recurrently. Women participation and reservation in the three tier panchayat system is a vital step to alleviate the inequality towards the women workers. The following recommendations should be considered by the policy makers in this regard:

o   Special attention should be given to the expansion of health insurance schemes such as RSBY and the same linked to programmes like ICDS, JSY, NRLM, NREGS & NULM, particularly benefitting the vulnerable and marginalized women.

o   A gender transformative health strategy which recognises women's reproductive rights should be develop and implemented.

o   The National Mental Health Policy (2014) recognises that women have a high risk of mental disorders due to various reasons like discrimination, violence and abuse. A systematic approach to provide requisite screening, care and treatment, especially primary level, should be developed.

o   Adult literacy with an added objective to link literacy programmes to life skills, financial literacy, and education on rights, law, and schemes, etc., in partnership with government schemes such as NRLM should be targeted.

o   Government should take initiatives to enhance the female education. The distance from school, especially secondary schools, is an important factor that impacts the enrolment and retention of girls in school, particularly in rural or remote areas. Improving the local transport system or free school bus services should be considered.

o   Gender wage gap across urban and rural, agriculture and non-agriculture, regular and casual jobs ahould be addressed to reduce discrimination.

o   The financial inclusion of women needs to be universalised so that women gain financial identity. The financial inclusion schemes should incorporate monitoring and evaluation mechanisms to assess gender equality and upliftment of the women belonging to the marginalised and vulnerable sectors.

o   Gender equity is an important concern for sustainable agricul-
     ture development. Efforts need to be made to support women
     farmers in their livelihood, ensure entitlements over agricultur-
     al services and provide social protection cover.

o   Skill development trainings for women should be developed to
     encourage them to take up forest-based, livestock-based, vege-
     table and agriculture based, poultry and fisheries based liveli-
     hood opportunities.

o   Women farmers or wives of farmers who committed suicide on
     account of failure of crop indebtedness are highly vulnerable
     and are left behind to take care of their children and family.
     Special packages for these women that contain comprehensive
     inputs of programmes of various department/ministries (like
     agriculture, rural development, KVIC, MWCD, etc.) should be
     provided to make them aware about the alternative livelihood
     options.

o   The service sector should encourage the equal employment op-
     portunities through jobs/enterprises for women especially in
     the high paid jobs.

o   Increasing the participation of women in civil services, judiciary
     and corporate entities should be targeted through appropriate
     modules for guidance and counselling, coaching, intensives and
     quotas.

15

Domestic Violence and Protection of Women

Nancy Prasanna Joseph

Abstract

Violence against women is a general scenario. While it varies in its degree from one society to the other, it prevails all over. The woman has consistently been subjected to violence on account of man. The crimes pertaining to women have existed constantly with time. The patterns of crime pertaining against her change with the adjustment in the outlook and procedures. The women are concurred a lower status in the public eye. From days of yore, women have been the ultimate recipients in the male-dominated society. The perplexing interactions of the powers of an inconsistent financial arrangement of the man-centric society produce a philosophy and worth framework, proliferating through a deceptive cycle of socialization and leading to auxiliary types of violence against women. Mistreatment and viciousness against women without a doubt have a social, mental, material, and sociological base. This chapter describes the domestic violence against women, the protection of women and the role of women policing in India.

Introduction

Domestic violence is the most widely recognized type of violence pertaining to women around the world, with 10 to 50% of women revealing corporal maltreatment by a marital partner in the course of their life. Consistently, brutality in the home and the society demolishes the lives of a large number of women. Around the globe, upwards of one out of three women had been battered, constrained into sex, or mishandled in a different way – more frequently by somebody she knows, including by her spouse or another male relative. On the other hand, one woman in four has been manhandled during pregnancy. Violence pertaining to women, be it in any structure, not just influences the women's wellbeing including their endurance, but on the other hand, is a danger factor for their long-term sickness.

Women perform an assortment of huge responsibility in our community since the birth till the end of their lives. In spite of performing all her jobs and entire activities in an effective manner in the contemporary world, a woman is tenuous as the society is still predominantly male-specific. Further, the life of a woman is more muddled than a man. She needs to deal with herself and relatives as a daughter, sister, spouse, mother, daughter-in-law, mother-in-law, granddaughter, grandmother, and so on.

The facts confirm that the last twenty years have seen exceptional human improvement endeavors contributing significantly in establishing women's abilities and in shutting gender inequalities. In spite of this advancement, a signiifcant imbalance among women and men exists with respect to the educational opportunities, well-being and nourishment.

In the pre-independent period, different endeavors have been carried out by the social reformers to inspire the status of women in India. The national movement initiated by Gandhi created an opportunity to achieve women advancements in social life. In India, the most recent decade has been set apart by the progression of the women's development. Emerging challenges have been elevated, new strategies are utilized for bringing mindfulness among women and various structures seem to activate women and voice their emotions and necessities. Indeed, the International Women's Decade emerged as a movement in India.

Status of Women in India

The status of a woman is a pugnacious subject in the present day society. The violence against women is a global issue. It influences women, all things considered, national groups, categorizations, and identities. It cuts across social and strict boundaries, blocking the privilege of women to partake completely in the public eye. Violence pertaining to women takes a disheartening assortment of structures, from family violence to assault, to childhood marriages, and to disfigurement. At the point when violence is submitted at home, it turns into domestic violence and includes relatives, for example, children, life partners, parents, or workers.

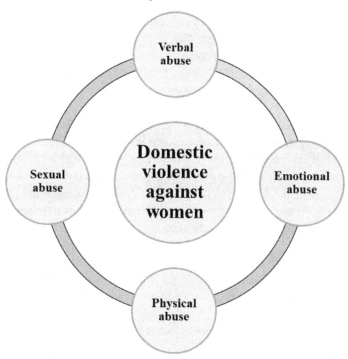

Figure 1. Domestic violence against women.

Figure 1 shows the the different abuses of domestic violence against women. Domestic violence is an aggressive behavior in the relationships that is utilized by one of the partners to pick up or keep up force and power over another marital partner. These behaviors include verbal, emotional, physical, and sexual abuse. Domestic violence can comprise of various methods, for example, beating, whipping, gnawing, pushing, controlling, tossing objects, etc. In more general terms, it incorporates threats, maltreatment, psychological mistreatment, domination or oppressive behavior, harassment, terrorization, clandestine maltreatment, financial hardship, assault, snatching, hijacking, murder, constraining wife or daughter-in-law to go for feticide, female feticide, compelling a widow of young age to perpetrate Sati, etc. The United Nations characterized "Violence against Women" in 1993 in Declaration on the Elimination of Violence against Women. It portrays it as an act of sex-based violence which causes physical, sexual, or emotional distress or torment to women. Each form of domestic violence constitutes the infringement of the most basic human rights.

India is famous for its social legacy, customs, progress, religion, and geological characteristics since olden days. On the contrary, it is also well known as a male dominated nation. The women in old days were restricted for domestic work. They were absolutely ignorant of their privileges and self-development.

Women constitute a large proportion of the population of the country, thus, the empowerment of women is vital. It is important to engage women to comprehend their privileges to be self-reliant in all fields for their development and progress. Women should be empowered as opposed to treating as a defenseless sufferer of male dominance. Along these lines, the government of India has started endless programs, plans, policies for women welfare.

Women's police stations are a special development that rose in postcolonial countries worldwide in the second half of the 20th century to handle violence pertaining to women. Violence pertaining to women is a worldwide problem, which affects all social orders. It abuses the rights and key opportunities of victims. Such violent activities can devastatingly affect the living conditions of victims, their families, and their communities. Thus, it is worthwhile to handle the violence against women by the women police.

Evolution of Police System and the Role of Women Police in India

The police institution is as old as the individual on the planet. The police power is needed to maintain the lawfulness. Traditionally, the police is considered as a male-dominated occupation. However, in the last few decades, various variables have contributed towards a more noteworthy acknowledgment of women in the police power. In spite of the fact that women entered the Indian police as early as 1938, their development and advancement have been moderate. Generally, women were utilized as social specialists as opposed to police officers, thus, managing matters concerning children and women. The women police power was actually built up in the year 1973 with one sub-inspector of police, one head constable, and 20 base staff. In the recent years, there has been an expansion in the number of women joining the Indian Police Service. Aside from standard work, there are women deputy superintendent of police in each locale.

Crime pertaining to women is a field of utmost need. Numerous steps have been embraced to handle this social danger. Firstly, particular emphasis has been given to counteract the violations against women by expanding police vigil and by strengthening the network. Further, restrictive All Women Police Stations (AWPSs) have been opened up in the states, and women helplines are working in subsequent AWPSs. The number of the women police has additionally been expanded extensively to address the issue.

Crimes pertaining to women defined under the Indian Penal Code (IPC) are:
- Molestation (Sec. 354 IPC)
- Domestic violence (Sec. 498A IPC)
- Sexual harassment (Sec. 509 IPC)
- Rape (Sec. 376 IPC)
- Cruelty by husband or relatives (Sec. 498-A IPC)
- Homicide for dowry, dowry deaths or their attempts (Sec. 302/304-B IPC)
- Kidnapping & abduction (Sec. 363- 373 IPC)
- Importation of girls (up to 21 years of age) (Sec. 366-B IPC)

The idea of All Women Police Stations solidified when it was understood that most of the crimes towards women had not been reported as a result of the hesitation of the women survivors to report the crime to the male-dominated police.

Commitment of Women Police

The significant commitment of women police has been in the field of tending to domestic violence confronted by women and assuming the function of an empathetic listener, guidance counselor, and adjuster. The Indian culture is one which esteems marriage as a consecrated foundation and assents women regard and position. Yet, incomprehensibly, there are no institutional systems to review the complaints of women confronting conjugal issues. The All Women Police Stations satisfy this crucial need.

Conclusion and Suggestions

The circumstances of many Indian women are very serious with respect of the brutality they suffer at home and outside. However, the awakening and knowledge among the women is leading to a change in this direction. The government policies have helped in overcoming this situation to some extent. Further, the role of women police in this direction is commendable and must be reinforced further.

References

Chakrabarti, S., & Biswas, C. S. (2012). An Exploratory analysis of women's empowerment in India: A Structural Equation Modelling Approach. Journal of Development Studies. https://doi.org/10.1080/00220388.2011.615920

Garcia-Moreno, C., Jansen, H. A., Ellsberg, M., Heise, L., & Watts, C. H. (2006). Prevalence of intimate partner violence: findings from the WHO multi-country study on women's health and domestic violence. Lancet. https://doi.org/10.1016/S0140-6736(06)69523-8

Gazmararian, J. A., Lazorick, S., Spitz, A. M., Ballard, T. J., Saltzman, L. E., & Marks, J. S. (1996). Prevalence of violence against pregnant women. In Journal of the American Medical Association. https://doi.org/10.1001/jama.275.24.1915

Heise, L., & García-Moreno, C. (2012). Violence By Intimate Partners. World Report on Violence and Health.

Howard, V. R. (2011). Gandhi's reconstruction of the feminine: Toward an indigenous hermeneutics. In Woman and Goddess in Hinduism: Reinterpretations and Re-envisionings. https://doi.org/10.1057/9780230119925_10

Ratanlal & Dhirajlal, The Indian Penal Code (2010). Lexis-Nexis India.

United Nations General Assembly. (1994). Declaration on the elimination of violence against women. In International Journal of Refugee Law. https://doi.org/10.1093/ijrl/6.4.714

16

Victim Shaming in Matters Concerning Sexual Offences in India and the Mandate of Developing Women Policing

Abhishek Rajesh Bhattacharjee
Shreya Das

Abstract

A country's growth depends on its people. The term 'people' includes both men and women of that particular society. Therefore, discrimination against anyone leads to a hindrance in the overall growth of the nation. A patriarchal society, which only believes in the good of its men, forgets that the non-upliftment of a major portion of its population, i.e. women, will not only lead to an immense stagnancy in the growth, but can also lead to an overall downfall of the society. Since time immemorial, society has always seen women as someone not having capabilities similar to that of men. They have been ill-treated and have also been prevented from enjoying equal rights as their counterparts. This problem not only extends to the national territorial limits, but has also got an international presence. Such a mindset is still prevalent in many societies. Time and again, people have been proved wrong due to the outstanding advancements made by the women. Respecting the choices made by women and not judging them based on such choices is very important. Their character is not defined by their way of life. People fail to understand that everyone has the right to choose his or her way of life which most of the times is taken away from women. Their character is assassinated based on their choices. This leads to injustice towards them, more so, when they are victims of sexual offences.

Research Objective

The endeavour is to show that the changes in the law concerning character evidence have played a significant role in initiating the process of elimination of the humiliation faced by a female victim in matters of sexual offences. The study incorporates a timeline of the various developments and an analysis concerning the 2013 amendment which can be considered to be a landmark modification in the domain of criminal law. The paper deals with the amendments made to the Indian Evidence Act, 1872, the Indian Penal Code, 1860 & the Code of Criminal Procedure, 1973 concerning character evidence and how these amendments have played a major role towards the elimination of discrimination against women. The scope is, hence, restricted to the domestic level. The paper ends with an extremely valuable recommendation which will ensure that the abolition of character assassination of victims gives the desired result.

Research Methodology

The researchers have chosen the problem with prodigious interest, keeping in mind its impelling and significant need in the present socio-legal conditions and circumstances. The method adopted to conduct the research is a doctrinal method accompanied with a qualitative analysis of the developments concerning the issue. Both primary as well as secondary sources are utilised to accumulate the relevant information. The material facts are collected from legal and non-legal sources like international legal instruments, books of legal experts of national and international repute, legislations, judgements, law journals, law reports, internet references and opinion of research scholars, academicians and other experts who have dealt with this subject.

Introduction

The character of a person in a matter, whether civil or criminal, plays a major role, and the intensity of the role is higher in criminal matters. Since time immemorial, the conduct and character of a person involved in a conflict have been of utmost importance in determining the actual aspects of that matter. This leads to a shift in concentration from the merits of the case to the less relevant and in many cases irrelevant aspect of character evidence. With time, many jurists have complained that judging a matter based on the character of either the victim or the accused deviates the concentration from the actual facts of the matter.

Both common law as well as the Indian law fail to provide an accurate definition of the term 'character evidence'. In the Indian context, character evidence is dealt with under sections 52 to 55 of the Indian Evidence Act, 1872. To understand the meaning of the term, one has to have a clear picture of the word 'character'. According to various dictionaries around the globe, the definition of character of a person can be narrowed down to the following points:

- A set of qualities in a person that make him/her different from others.
- A particular quality of a person as described by others.
- The difference in the behaviour of a person from that of others, especially in a way that is interesting.

Normally, in any case, it is only the character of the accused which is considered to be relevant and is given a high degree of importance by the judiciary. Although, the relevancy concerning the issue of the case has to be established separately, however, there was an exception made to this rule whereby the character of the victim was taken into consideration in determining the issue concerning the consent of the victim or the quality of that consent in matters related to outraging the modesty of a woman and sexual offences. The victim, who already had to go through a lot of trauma, was again made to face irrelevant questions by the investigators trying to assassinate her character to change the direction of the case.

Sexual Offences Under the Indian Penal Code

Sexual offences against women have been dealt with under section 354, section 354A-D, section 376 and section 376A-E of the IPC[1]. The motive behind enacting section 354 of the Indian Penal Code, 1860 was to safeguard a woman against improper assault and protect her morality. The constituents or the ingredients which determine outraging a woman's modesty are nowhere defined. These differ according to the facts and circumstances of a particular case and according to the present moral, social and legal ethics of the country. In the case of *Pandurang Mahale v. State of Maharashtra*[2], the term modesty had been dealt with as a virtue attached to a female owing to her gender. Even if modesty is likely to be outraged due to any act, then the same shall also constitute an offence. A clear definition of modesty had been given in the case of *Ramkripal v. State of MP*[3]

---

[1] The Indian Penal Code, 1860 (Act 45 of 1860).
[2] AIR 2004 SC 1677.
[3] (2007) 11 SCC 265.

whereby the apex court held: *"The essence of a woman's modesty is her gender. The act of pulling a woman, removing her saree, coupled with a request of sexual nature...would be an outrage to the modesty of a woman; and knowledge, that modesty is likely to be outraged, is sufficient to constitute the offence."* Sections 354A, 354B, 354C and 354D[4] have been incorporated by the Criminal Law (Amendment) Act, 2013, which has added various spectrums to the concept of outraging a women's modesty such as sexual harassment, assaulting a woman with the motive to disrobe, voyeurism and stalking, etc.

A major change was brought about by amendment concerning the punishment for rape whereby the punishment was to be given based on the gravity of the offence committed. Earlier, section 376 only dealt with the punishment of rape whereby a punishment for a period of maximum 7 years along with fine could be imposed. However, it was with the amendment that various avenues to section 376 were incorporated and the punishment was to be awarded based on the severity of those avenues on a case to case basis. Sections 376A, 376B, 376C, 376D and 376E were added to give a broader view to the aspect of rape[5]. Punishments were laid down for causing death or resulting in a persistent vegetative state of the victim, sexual harassment by a husband with his wife during separation, sexual harassment by a person holding certain authority and repeat offenders.

Relevance of Character of Victim Before 2013

Earlier, the character of a victim was taken into consideration while determining cases regarding sexual offences against women. One of the biggest examples is the case of *Tukaram and Anr v. State of Maharashtra*[6] which is commonly referred to as the Mathura rape case. It was a clear example of denial of justice to the victim based on illogical and baseless reasoning. Without paying any heed to the merits of the case, it was the character of the victim which was continuously questioned and attacked. This led to protests among the masses which ultimately led to the enactment of the Criminal Law

---

[4] *Supra* note 1.
[5] *Ibid.*
[6] 1979 (2) SCC 143.

(Amendment) Act of 1983. Section 114A of the Evidence Act[7] was amended, and it was laid down that it shall be presumed by any court dealing with a case of a sexual offence against women that the victim did not have consent. Section 376 of the IPC[8] was also amended whereby custodial rape was made punishable with punishment up to a period of 7 years. The burden of proving the same was also shifted from the victim to the offender.

The character assassination of a victim while questioning her in the process of cross-examination also increases the mental agony and pain of the victim. The amendments made in the Mathura case did not help the cause. In many cases, this was used as an armour to safeguard the culprits from any kind of punishment. Though in cases like *Sakshi v. Union of India and ors.[9]*, the court laid measures to curb this menace, but an alteration of the provisions was still required to completely stop the process. Earlier the law was such that during cross-examination, a victim could be put to any questions. Her past relationships and her past sexual encounters were put before her as questions, thereby, leading to severe emotional strain. Though the protection against these types of questions during the process of cross-examination was provided by the Indian Evidence (Amendment) Act, 2002, the same was not complete as the ambit of rape was very much constrained. The provisions had to undergo another amendment to incorporate the broader aspects of rape enacted by the 2013 Amendment.

However, even after many changes made to various acts and countless steps taken to make the system proper, the character assassination was still seen in the Nirbhaya case[10] of 2012. The modern and western lifestyle of the victim and the fact that she was an independent professional were considered to be 'invitations' for sexual assault. Everyone failed to understand that the evil of rape did not occur due to the choices made by the victim but it occurred due to the mindset of the culprits. The protests and mass uprising led to the passing of the Criminal Law (Amendment) Act, 2013 whereby section 53A was added under the topic of character evidence in the

---

[7] The Indian Evidence Act, 1872 (Act 1 of 1872).
[8] *Supra* note 5.
[9] (2004) 5 SCC 518.
[10] (2017) 3 SCC 717.

Evidence Act; the proviso to section 146 was also substituted in the Act and it was stated that evidence of the character of the victim regarding the person's previous sexual experience shall not be considered to be relevant during the process of cross-examination.[11] The victim cannot be made to face questions regarding her previous sexual experience and general immoral character to determine whether she consented or not. This was a major change which was brought about to curb the menace of character assassination prevalent in the system and because of which the focus of the case always shifted from the merits of the case.

Changes Made Via 2013 Amendment and Present Scenario

The three major changes brought about, pertaining to the relevance of the character of the women in case of a sexual offence were the inscription of section 53A, amendment made to section 114A and the amendment made to section 146 in the Indian Evidence Act, 1872.[12] The major revolution was brought about by the incorporation of section 53A which formulated that in cases of sexual offences, where the consent of the victim is an issue, the previous sexual experiences of the victim with any other person shall not be taken into consideration in determining such consent or quality of such consent. Generally, in criminal cases, it is the character of the accused which is considered to be relevant under section 53 of the Indian Evidence Act, 1872 to conclude a matter. However, section 53A which was incorporated through the 2013 amendment specifically deals with the character of the victim and the fact that it would not play any role whatsoever in determining whether the victim had given her consent in cases of sexual offences. Whether the victim is married or non-married, whether the victim has been into any previous sexual relationships or not, etc., won't be a determining factor when the issue regarding her consent in a given case concerning sexual offence is being looked into. The entire purpose of this particular incorporation is to prevent the character assassination of the victim which was visible in several cases. When the character of a female, who has been a victim of such a horrendous crime, is further murdered during the investigation as well as during the judicial processs, it becomes much more traumatising for the person at the

---

[11] *Supra.* Note 7.
[12] *Ibid.*

receiving end which leads to the victim getting highly scared & embarrassed. The existing scenario defeated the purpose of justice as the merits of the case were not looked into. Moreover, proper and complete truth could not be deciphered as the person who could reveal the same had to face utmost mental agony and emotional pain which prevented her from revealing the same. Section 53A also laid the inception of the arena that the consent at the first instance cannot be considered to be consent in the second instance too.

The second vital change brought about was the substitution of section 114A with a new one whereby in rape matters, falling under the ambit of clauses a to n of section 376(2) of the Indian Penal Code, 1860, the court was mandated to presume the absence of consent of the victim. This implied that the history of the personal life of the victim cannot influence the decision of the court on the issue of consent of the victim in any given case. The third and final change was the inscription of a new section 146 whereby it is provided that the act of collecting evidence regarding the general immoral character of the victim to establish the consent of the victim is not permissible at all. Similarly, the act of asking questions regarding the previous sexual experiences to the victim is also disallowed to determine the issue of consent as all these leads to embarrassment for the victim, which may prevent the truth from being revealed.

Some major changes were also brought about in the Indian Penal Code, 1860 which ensures that the victim does not have to go through the trauma of character assassination after the horrendous incident has already occurred with her. According to the amendments made in the year 2013, section 166A has been added to the Indian Penal Code, 1860 which penalises the public servants who refuse to record the first information report in specified crimes against women. In this amendment, the term 'consent' was also given a proper definition by adding an explanation to section 375 of the Indian Penal Code, 1860. The term is defined as an unequivocal voluntary agreement which signifies the willingness of the woman by the use of words, gestures, and any form of verbal or non-verbal communications. The definition makes the fact crystal clear that a woman's silence cannot be considered to be a yes. The punishment was also included for the rape conducted by a man on his wife during the period of separation which was previously missing.

The various provisions regarding the processes of recording the first information report, recording of the statement of the victim by the judicial magistrate, when the crime is committed by a public servant and provisions for free medical help by public/private hospitals under the Code of Criminal Procedure, 1973 were also amended to make things much easier for the victim. These changes were to make sure that the victim does not face any kind of character assassination after she had to go through so much. These steps were very much necessary to eliminate the discrimination which was rampant against the victims and survivors of sexual offences based on their previous choices made in life.

The consent of a female cannot be construed to be present in a case of sexual offences even if the female is a sex worker. This is a very important fact which can be very well interpreted from the changes brought about by the amendments made in the year 2013. The various process of cross-examination, recording of a first information report, recording of statements of the victim, etc., shall be same even if the victim's profession is that of a sex worker. Working as a sex worker is not a tag that automatically signifies or denotes consent when such an act is committed.

Development of Women Policing – The Way Forward

It is beyond doubt that the altered laws have initiated the process of eliminating the hardships faced by a female victim while seeking justice in matters concerning sexual offences. However, the motive behind the modifications will not be fulfilled in its entirety until and unless there is a change in the ground reality. Even today, many victims of such heinous crimes think more than twice before going to the police station to lodge a complaint against the injustice on the ground that her previous sexual encounters or lifestyle will be questioned and laughed upon by the male dominated police department. The women are scared to reveal the details of the unfortunate and barbaric act to the male police officers. This is where women police officials play a very significant role.

Justice fails to prevail in matters concerning sexual offences till the details of the matter are unearthed to the core. To increase the chances of excavating intricate information in such cases so that appropriate justice is served on an urgent basis, it is very much necessary that the comfortability factor of the victim is increased to such a level that she can open up more freely. This will not only initiate speedy disposal of such matters but will also ensure that justice is served to all. Today, more than half of the cases concerning molestation and rape are not reported due to the sole reason that the victim is not comfortable to share her trauma in totality with a male police officer.

Therefore, to ensure that the objectives behind the amendments are carried out fully, development of women policing is a mandate. A significant increase in the number of female recruits in the police department is the need of the hour. Only then, more victims will come forward to seek justice, and the perpetrators who are roaming freely will face appropriate consequences under the law.

Conclusion

Even after many changes brought about in the criminal justice system, the discrimination against the women at the receiving end of the sexual offences is not completely eradicated from the society. People need to understand that our constitution guarantees us the right to live our lives in our own way, provided that in doing so we do not hamper the rights of the others. This is similar for both the genders of the society. While the male counterpart of the society is not discriminated based on the choices made by him, it is a very astonishing fact that the female counterparts are always hunted down by making such discriminations. The patriarchal mindset of the people stops them from acknowledging the fact that a woman can lead her life at her own terms, and she has all the capabilities to do so in an independent manner.

When a woman faces a horrendous sexual crime or when her modesty is outraged by any means, it leaves a dent on her mind and soul along with the wounds on her body. Some of the victims get so frightened and embarrassed that they even tend to end their lives. A woman's way of life and her choices are held responsible for the heinous acts inflicted upon her. People forget that it is not due to the choice of a female that she has to face such a thing but it is the backward and vulgar mindset of the wrongdoers due to which the act has occurred.

Before the 2013 alterations, there was a failure to get hold of the correct facts which made sure that the wrongdoers are not punished properly (and in certain cases are not punished at all). However, no amendment can make sure that such kind of discrimination is eliminated until and unless the people of the society at large understand the fact that it is not the choice of any woman but the mindset of the culprits which gives rise to such horrendous crimes. The backing of the society and media is very much essential to revive the confidence in the survivors/victims and make sure that their right to justice prevails. They should be made to feel that their choices, their previous sexual encounters, their way of life, their dressing style, etc., are not responsible for the crime committed on them. Until and unless this is not ensured, the present system of justice cannot work to its full potential.

Moreover, to certify the implementation of the alteration at the ground level, developing the scenario of women policing in the country is of utmost importance. The development will increase the comfortability factor in the victims and will enable them to speak about the atrocities without any hesitation while filing a complaint at the police station. It will ensure that more victims come forward to seek justice, and their faith in the police department is restored.

17

Participation of Women in Indian Police

Muskan Jain
Bhupal Bhattacharya

Abstract

Police system is the most important executory body of a nation, and it must represent diversity in terms gender, race, ethnicity, religion, etc., in its representation to society. In this chapter, we are going to analyze this diversity in terms of gender and participation of women in police system in Indian scenario. Although the importance of women police is accepted throughout the world on various aspects, yet, the participation in India is still 7.28%. There are different reasons and causes for low participation, but one of the major root causes is the concept of patriarchal values and mindset. This chapter also deals with other causes like prejudiced attitude towards women, unequal and discriminatory distribution of work, poor facilities and sexual harassment at workplace. Despite many guidelines issued by central government, we are way back in promoting equal, friendly and secure workplace for females in police force as the first step to eradicate this problem is to end the patriarchy, which is very challenging to achieve.

Introduction

India is the land of one of the oldest civilizations and has evolved gradually with the principles of patriarchy in its system. The nation is also built upon the religious practices and customs. More precisely, it does not focus on a single religion, rather it is a home of diverse religious customs and values[1]. The concept of patriarchy in India has divided the professions on the basis of their gender. It has been evolved as a great belief that police is a masculine profession and females are not made for it[2].

India has faced the problem of gender discrimination over time and on different occasions. We bring many legislations and constitutional amendments to give equal rights to the women, but patriarchy has deepened its roots in our society so much that we even do not realize when we become the part of it[3]. We cannot blame any particular section for the problem of gender discrimination as it is a social evil and we ourselves are society.

Our society has divided the professions on the basis of gender. In this respect, police is considered as a profession which needs physical strength[4]. There may be some other reasons, like religious restrictions, which also restrict females. To provide equality and equal opportunities to women, our Constitution has many provisions. For instance, Article 14 provides right to equality; Article 15 provides no discrimination on the ground of caste, colour, race and sex; Article 16 provides equal opportunities regardless of any discrimination on the grounds of caste, religion, race and sex; and Article 39(d) provides for equal pay for equal work[5]. Apart from the Constitution, there are several legislations which safeguard the interest of women in various sectors[6]. Along with the national laws, India has signed various international treaties which make it an obligation to provide equal status to women, like Universal Declaration of Human Rights (UDHR), the Convention on the Elimination of all forms of Discrimination Against Women (CEDAW), the International Covenant on Civil and Political Rights (ICCPR), etc[7]. However, the legislations and constitutional provisions are only helpful if there is a significant participation of women in professional aspects.

According to a report, participation of women in police is only 7.28% of the total police. In India, more than 20 states have reservations for women, ranging from 4% to 38% in police services. Still, their total participation is less than 10%. Out of 7.28% of women police, almost 89.37% are at constabulary position, 9.76% are at the rank of investigators and only 0.85% are at the supervisory position[8]. This reflects two scenarios of our police system for females. Firstly, the participation of women in the police is insignificant and secondly, the women police are excluded from the major roles. The reasons for the prevailing situation are explained below.

Causes of Insignificant Participation

There are several reasons of gender bias in police force which may include working conditions for female staff, concept of patriarchy, attitude towards female police, sexual harassment at workplace, etc.

Strong belief in patriarchy

It is a very strong belief and a mindset that the police services belong to the males of the society and it is a masculine profession, which needs a lot of physical strength and emotional stability, which are lacking in a female[9]. It is a very adamant and a stubborn pledge towards patriarchy. As we know, it took us decades to arrive at the onset of women empowerment by substituting some values of the prevailing patriarchy. However, it is still affected by the male chauvinism and deep-rooted old practices. The classical example of this incident is India's first woman IPS officer, Kiren Bedi. When Kiran Bedi cleared her examination, she was denied an appointment as an IPS officer on the grounds of her gender. She approached the Supreme Court and demanded justice as it violated her fundamental rights of equality. The Supreme Court allowed her appointment, however, she was deliberately posted in Tihar Jail in Delhi, which houses the most dangerous criminals. She accepted the challenge, and transformed the jail. For her efforts, she was awarded by Raman Magsaysay Award. Overall, it is still believed by the system that females are incapable of handling the cases of high intensity; and they should give priority to their home instead of police force.

Working conditions

Distribution of tasks: It has been observed through various surveys and discussions that female officers are basically assigned in-home tasks like maintaining registers, data management, dealing with general public, filing NCR or FIR reports, etc., and they are not assigned for field visits and works like patrolling, maintaining law and order, investigations, enquiry, etc. These tasks are assigned to the male officers. As discussed earlier, around 90% of the female police personnel are at the rank of constables and doing the clerical work. Major gaps between the tasks of the male and female officers is observed in Delhi and Bihar. In contract, Nagaland and Punjab have shown greater proportions of women police in the field work.

Duty hours and weekly off: Though, a female is doing the same work as her husband or any male member of her family, she has to additionally manage her household and children single handedly. In police services, the duty hours and weekly holidays are inappropriate in maintaining the balance with the domestic work of policewomen. According to a report, almost 48% women have reported no weekly off, and around 29% of women get a day off in a week.

This situation is worse in the states like Orissa and Chhattisgarh, where it has been reported respectively by 90 and 95% women police that they do not get any weekly off. Apart from the weekly holidays, women police also had to stay back after their duty due to increasing work load, insufficient staff, emergency needs, etc. Around 18% females registered emergency duties as their main cause of overtime, and 29% registered too much workload as the main cause.

Separate sanitation facilities: Improper and inadequate sanitation facilities are one of the major reasons of low women participation in many of the professions, and police system is one of them. The police stations are still facing the lack of women toilets or inadequate sanitation facilities. On average, 22% of female officers have reported that they do not have the access to separate toilets at their workplace. 61% female police in Bihar and 59% in Telangana reported the same. In this regard, Delhi is the best performing state, with separate toilets for 99% women police staff.

Attitude towards female police
Discrimination and inequality: The work environment of the police job is not considered to be friendly for females, rather is very discriminatory[10]. As discussed earlier, the females are devoid of appropriate promotions and distribution of work. They are assigned the 'in-house' tasks like maintaining registers, data, etc., and they are not assigned field jobs like investigations. Less than 10% of the total women force is at supervisory level, and they are mostly appointed at constable level. Bihar, Jharkhand and West Bengal are known to have significant discrimination towards women.

Preconception and sexism towards women: Traditionally, holding all the patriarchal views, the police profession is considered to be a masculine occupation, and females are not deemed fit to work in this environment[11]. It is believed that women are incapable of fulfilling their duties as police officer and will have to do compromises because of their lack of physical strength, emotional and sensitive being and domestic responsibilities[12].

Sexual harassment at workplace
Sexual harassment at workplace or casting couch is a common syndrome of every occupation. It is the most devastating hindrance in actual women empowerment. A minimal or no implementation of

Sexual Harassment Act, 2013 for having a sexual harassment committee at every workplace is noted.

Need of Women in Police

Police system is a workplace which requires diverse recruitment, in terms of gender as well as ethnicity. In a country like India, which is known for its diversity, it becomes even more vital[13]. There are numerous examples where women have proved themselves in different fields of work[14]. The following are the reasons for the need of women in police:

Accomplished in addressing gender based crimes

Around the globe, we are facing a drastic increase in gender based crimes, be it rape, sexual harassment, domestic violence, dowry deaths, eve-teasing, acid attacks, etc[15]. However, a majority of the real incidents go unreported and majority of the reported incidents are false. The National Family Health Survey (NFHS) report of 2015-16 reveals that 99% of cases of sexual harassment go unreported. There are many reasons for not recording these incidents which come into play, such as, fear of social stigma, suspicions in police employees[16].

This particular area of police services majorly requires the involvement and recruitment of women police, as women can embark a major change in this scenario. Secondly, sexual offences are very intimate for a female victim, and a woman police can play a vital role in handling these. The victim might open more securely to a female officer, rather than to a male officer. As per a report, "Data from 39 countries shows that the presence of women police officers correlates positively with reporting of sexual assault, which confirms that recruiting women is an important component of a gender-responsive justice system".

Minimum use of excessive power

It is true to an extent that women are less probable to use force and wrench out their weapons. They do not lose their cool easily and are more stable in their anger levels. Indeed, police requires more aggression and physical strength, but there are many situations when use of force does not work. This is specifically important during the time when the use of force by a police officer is under increased scrutiny, often causing intensified tensions between police and the societies they serve. National Centre for Women and Policing report of 2010 states that *"twenty years of exhaustive research demonstrates that women police officers utilize a style of policing that relies less on physical force, and more on communication skills that defuse potentially violent situations. Women police officers are therefore much less likely to be involved in occurrences of police brutality, and are also much more likely to effectively respond to police calls regarding violence against women."*

Developing better police-community relations

A sheriff detective of San Diego, Tiffany Townsend, said, "The dedication to ethical conduct and compassionate service is what law enforcement is, or should be, all about." Law enforcement is a public service which requires a very peaceful and humble relationship between the police and public. It is very important for public to trust their officers. It has been observed that female police is less authoritarian in their attitude towards public, which is essential for maintaining the harmony with the communities and public. Most notably, the female officers are better at resolving possibly violent confrontations *before* those encounters which turn deadly.

What is Needed to be Done?

In India, the subject matters and power over them are defined under Constitution, and police system is the subject matter which comes under state jurisdiction. Hence, the state governments have the power to make rules associated with the police. The union government from time to time issues guidelines for proper functioning of the system, however, these are not binding over state governments[17]. This is the basic reason that the situation of the female police varies from state to state.

The union government, in 2009, set a benchmark of at least 33% female representation in police services, but only union territories and nine states (Andhra Pradesh, Jharkhand, Gujarat, Maharashtra, Madhya Pradesh, Nagaland, Odisha, Telangana and Tamil Nadu) have accepted and implemented this benchmark. Further, the union government advised in 2013 that there must be at least 3 sub-inspector and at least 10 female constables in every police station. It was proposed by the union government in 2015 that Investigative

Units for Crimes against Women (IUCAW) must at least comprise of 1/3rd of female staff in every crime-prone district[18-26].

Above all, it is vital to maintain a balance between the tasks and responsibilities assigned to men and women, along with providing equal opportunities of promotion to females. In addition, a dignified environment is needed to be maintained so that a woman feels secure to join the police force. It is also important to spread awareness through educational institutions and media platforms to motivate more female candidates to opt for police as their profession.

Overall, the prevailing challenges can be overcome through proper implementation of laws and codes of conduct to eliminate the sexual harassment, gender based discrimination and patriarchal mindset.

References

1. Lerner, G. (1986). *The creation of patriarchy* (Vol. 1). Oxford University Press, USA.
2. Huyer, S., & Sikoska, T. (2003). *Overcoming the gender digital divide: understanding ICTs and their potential for the empowerment of women.* Santo Domingo: INSTRAW.
3. Cook, R. J. (Ed.). (2012). *Human rights of women: National and international perspectives.* University of Pennsylvania Press.
4. Rabe-Hemp, C. E. (2009). POLICE women or police WOMEN? Doing gender and police work. *Feminist criminology, 4*(2), 114-129.
5. Sullivan, K. M. (2002). Constitutionalizing Women's Equality. *Calif. L. Rev., 90,* 735.
6. Hellum, A., & Aasen, H. S. (Eds.). (2013). *Women's human rights: CEDAW in international, regional and national law* (Vol. 3). Cambridge University Press.
7. Cook, R. J., & World Health Organization. (1994). *Women's health and human rights: the promotion and protection of women's health through international human rights law.* World Health Organization.
8. Biddle, K., Clegg, I., & Whetton, J. (1999). Evaluation of ODA/DFID support to the police in developing countries: A synthesis study. *Swansea: Centre for Development Studies.*

Available at:< URL: http://www. swan. ac. uk/cds/pdffiles, 20.

9. Bouza, A. V. (2013). *The police mystique: An insider's look at cops, crime, and the criminal justice system.* Springer.

10. Scanlon, M. C. T. N. T., & Dworkin, R. (1977). *Equality and preferential treatment.* Princeton University Press.

11. Meier, M. M. (2013). " Doing Gender" or" Doing Policing?" Gender Identity and Gender Role Beliefs Among Police Officers.

12. Lemelle Jr, A. J. (2010). *Black masculinity and sexual politics* (Vol. 2). Routledge.

13. Hakim, C. (1996). *Key issues in women's work: Female heterogeneity and the polarisation of women's employment* (Vol. 4). A&C Black.

14. Waters, I., Hardy, N., Delgado, D., & Dahlmann, S. (2007). Ethnic minorities and the challenge of police recruitment. *The Police Journal, 80*(3), 191-216.

15. Babu, D. (2019). Gender Based Violence in India: An Analysis of National Level Data for Theory, Research and Prevention.

16. Kirschman, E. (2018). *I love a cop: What police families need to know.* Guilford Publications.

17. Goldberg, C. E. (1974). Public Law 280: The Limits of State Jurisdiction over Reservation Indians. *UCLA L. Rev., 22,* 535.

18. Data on Police Organisations as on 01.01.2017, Bureau of Police Research and Development, Ministry of Home Affairs, Government of India, pg. 152-153.

19. Bureau of Police Research and Development, Ministry of Home Affairs, 'Data on Police Organizations (Report 2017)' Available at <http://bprd.nic.in/WriteReadData/userfiles/ file/databook2017.pdf> [Last accessed on 13 July 2019]

20. Government of India, Ministry of Home Affairs, Advisory (2015),15011/72/2014 – SC/ST – W : https://mha.gov.in/sites/default/files/CrimesagainstWom en0601.PDF

21. Government of India, Ministry of Home Affairs, Advisory (2013), D.O.No.15011/21 – SC/ST – W:https://mha.gov.in/sites/default/files/AdvisoryWomenP olice-290513.pdf

22. Bhattacharya, P. and Kundu, T. , 2018, '99% cases of sexual assaults go unreported, govt data shows' , Livemint, 24 April. Available at <https://www.livemint.com/Politics/ AV3sIKoEBAGZozALMX8THK/99-cases-of-sexual-assaults-

go-unreported-govt-data-shows.html> [Last accessed on 27 July 2019].

23. Human Rights Watch, '"Everyone Blames Me" Barriers to Justice and Support Services for Sexual Assault Survivors in India (Report 2017). Available at <https://www.hrw.org/ sites/default/files/report_pdf/india1117_web.pdf>   [Last accessed on 3 July 2019].

24. United Nations Women report in 2011-'12 titled "Progress of the World's Women: In Pursuit of Justice".

25. National Centre for Women and Policing, (website homepage) http://womenandpolicing.com

26. Common Cause–Centre for the Study of Developing Societies, 'Status of Policing in India Report (SPIR 2018)'. Available at <https://www.lokniti.org/media/upload_files/ Report%20Police%20Survey.pdf> [Last accessed on 14 July 2019].

18

Role of Women Police Stations in Combatting Crimes in India in the 21st Century

Shibasish Bhattacharjee
Ankita Sen

Abstract

In India, the women entered the police force not before early 1938, however, their growth and development in the department have been slow, yet steady. In the early years, women were seen more in the role of social workers of the justice department, focused on issues pertaining to broadly women and children. However, due to advancement in the field of education and literacy, in the 21st century, people across the country and the world have understood the requirement of women in the policing services. In the past few decades, India has been a witness to a large number of women joining the Indian Police Services (IPS). India has devised and implemented steady mechanisms to inculcate more females into the profession of policing. However, more needs to be done to enhance the participation of women in the police service.

Introduction

The police organisations in India are on a mission to adopt all measures to eliminate any sort of disparity towards women. Like any other institution governed by the state, every individual police unit needs to adhere to the right of equality, practice the art of non-discrimination and provide equality of opportunity as given by the Constitution of India. The Preamble guarantees all the citizens to an equality of opportunity and status (Article 14 (Equality before law), Article 15 (Prohibition of discrimination on the grounds of religion, race caste, sex, place of birth) and Article 16 (Equality in matters of public employment)). Such rights not only glorify the right to equality in a broader perspective, but also make provisions for special laws. For instance, Article 15 allows the state to make special provisions in matter of governance of children and women, among other vulnerable groups. The acceptance of the facts that women's emancipation and growth has been cut off due to societal stratification, and it is the responsibility of the institutions of the state[1] to take appropriate and immediate measures to cover up this disparity, is vital. Such obligation is heightened by India's commitment internationally to attain gender equality, and the betterment of women is a central aim of the government, aimed at advancing, strengthening and entitling women.

The Commonwealth Human Rights Initiative (CHRI)[2] is a vital initiative to attain human rights, genuine democracy and development. CHRI enshrines these values through planned thoughts and standing up for human rights, access to justice and access to information. It does so through research, publications, workshops, information dissemination and advocacy. In many nations, the police are seen as an oppressive instrument of state rather than as protectors of citizens' rights, leading to widespread refusal of rights and no access to the wheels of justice. CHRI promotes a systemic reform so that the police act as bearers of the rule of law rather than as tools of the current regime. In India, CHRI's programme aims at utilizing, public support for police reform. In South Asia, CHRI works to strengthen the society engagement on police reforms. In East Africa and Ghana, CHRI has examined the police accountability issues and political interference. CHRI has a plan to make the prison systems effective, where the treatment of the prisoners would be more transparent.

Bhartiya Stree Shakti (BSS)

The Bhartiya Stree Shakti was founded in 1988. It is a participatory and voluntary organisation without any political ties, working towards the issues of gender equality, economic independence and education of women. This organisation is rooted for shaping the lives of women and their families, but also taking care of the health issues, financial independence, thus, boosting their self-esteem and morale. Their aim is to make the women independent and focused, thus, making them stand on their own feet and emancipating them from the patriarchal bondages. BSS is a notable and sought after non-governmental pioneer aimed at verifying and reviewing policies, creating mass awareness and engaging with the central and state government employees. Many initiatives have been successfully put in action, to

---

[1] https://indiankanoon.org/search/?formInput=state%20law
[2] https://www.humanrightsinitiative.org/content/careers

provide much required validation and suggestions with respect to the government policies.

The Bhartiya Stree Shakti[3] has played a poignant role in bringing information about the various government benefits and initiatives aimed specifically at women. A primary objective of the "National Policy for Women, 2016"[4] is to alienate and eradicate all forms of torture against women, through implementing improved and sustainable policies, firm legislations and programmes. The Nirbhaya case[5] was an eye-opener. At the onset of this incident, there was a significant outburst of protests and agitations by the general public, which led to the establishment of a judicial committee to study the most appropriate ways to reform the laws and to conduct swift investigations. In 2013, the then President of India, Mr. Pranab Mukherjee, disseminated the Criminal Law (Amendment) Bill[6], where several new legislations and bylaws were passed, and six new fast track courts were set up to try rape cases.

The violence against women is a challenge to the policing system and the society. With a steady increase in the different crimes committed against women, a serious introspection is needed into the cause of such an increase in the violence.

Violence Against Women, Police and Policing

The acts of violence against women include the physical, sexual and psychological abuse, including pounding, abuse of female children in the house, violence pertaining to dowry, marital rape[7], female genital mutilation[8] and other orthodox practices which are harmful to women. Such acts also include forced abortion, coercive use of contraceptives, female birth killings and prenatal sex determination. The violence involving adolescent and young girls predominantly includes child abuse, female foeticide, prostitution and flesh trading.

---

[3] http://www.bharatiyastreeshakti.org/
[4] https://wcd.nic.in/acts/draft-national-policy-women-2016
[5] https://www.bbc.com/news/world-asia-india-51969961
[6] https://indiankanoon.org/doc/544006/
[7] https://harvardhrj.com/2019/01/marital-rape-a-non-criminalized-crime-in-india/
[8] https://www.who.int/news-room/fact-sheets/detail/female-genital-mutilation

Women are challenged to face a wide range of obstacles in their attempts, not only while accessing the government services, but on a broader perspective. Though the representation of women in the high profile jobs has statistically grown, however, more needs to be done in this regard. If we see in the broader perspective, across the world, women are not represented equally in law enforcement. There has been a need to even the playing field by inducting women into this profession. At the same time, a system of checks and balances is needed to be established to improve deterrence of crimes against women. In this respect, the government and police need to take measures to actively prevent crimes against women and society as a whole. A viable solution to this problem is to formulate innovative ways in which women can be a part of the system, for instance, establishing "all women police stations" (WPS).

Effectiveness of Measures of Deterrence

It can be assumed that women police stations[9] can help in tackling gender-based violence, as the creation of such stations is targeted for the female victims. It has been seen in 19 odd states that after the implementation of women police stations, arrests arising due to female kidnapping cases have gone up by 15 percent. Such increments are important, in lieu of the fact that developing women's access to justice is not a conclusive evidence to prevent crimes committed against females. Prevention of such offences is also vitally needed. For instance, the women police stations in Tamilnadu are evenly distributed in the state and are at par with the women-controlled police stations in the United States.

The Effectiveness of Gender Responsive Policing (GRP)

Gender responsive interventions are deeply embedded in the socio-cultural background and are bound to be affected by the context. Due to dearth of information on the effectiveness of intercessions, the below discussion briefly describes the realms of attaining feasibility to implement different GRP[10] intercessions in South Asia. Such common GRP intercessions are:

---

[9] http://www.kolkatapolice.gov.in/section.asp?PSID=98&Typ=PS
[10] https://www.unwomen.org/en/digital-library/publications/2021/01/handbook-gender-responsive-police-services

Community policing[11]: There has been sufficient evidence available from South Asia, about the financial capacity of implementing community policing interventions and also the practicality of it for improving gender alertness. Taking into account the lack of trust, the idea of community policing would reduce the gap between the police and community as a whole.

Training and sensitization: The key skill of the GRP interjections is training. As the police society in India and in most countries is heavily male-dominated, training with a clear focus and aspiration to change one's attitude is highly required.

Women police stations: There has been a large number of women police stations established all over the world, especially in South Asia, and on account of which there has been a dramatic increase in the reporting of gender-based violence issues. On the other hand, an increasing number of cases have been solved too. It has to be noted that women police in the WPS have to time and again undergo rigorous training in order to upgrade themselves.

Special police cells: It has been observed that establishing special police units in South Asia has led to the recording of a high number of cases regarding gender-based crimes. Commonly, these special cells[12] are located inside the local police stations, and it is the duty of the police and government to raise awareness among the community.

One stop centres[13]: Such centres were first established in Africa. These centres aim at providing services related to justice, health, psycho-social support, thus, incentivizing women to join such centres. The biggest challenges include setting such a system and skilled labour for providing services.

Community policing has been an aspiring GRP intercession which has instilled confidence among women, along with changing the behaviour and approach of the police. It has also reduced apathy towards the police stations, leading to more cases being reported and filed.

---

[11] https://www.everbridge.com/blog/what-is-community-policing/
[12] https://tiss.edu/view/11/projects/all-projects/special-cell-for-women-and-children-maharashtra/
[13] https://wcd.nic.in/schemes/one-stop-centre-scheme-1

Training/sensitization of police is a common GRP intervention and is used mostly with other interventions. It is an essential subdivision of the other GRP interventions. Studies have reported that training is successful in improving knowledge, attitude and training of police workforce while dealing with the cases of gender based violence (GBV)[14]. Gender sensitive training is helpful to reconciliate the growing gender bias and cultural practices in police personnel. However, constant efforts, with repeated follow ups, are needed to retain the changed attitudes in the police. The women are satisfied with the services provided at the all-women police stations. Thus, the all-women police stations have become a massive success, fulfilling their objective. Special units further boost reporting of cases of women related violence. One stop centre is also an aspiring initiative to provide a plethora of services to victims of hatred. The centres that provide such services at hospitals, increase the efficiency of the process by manifolds.

The police are a subject under the purview of the state government, as laid down in the Constitution[15]. The central government has the autonomy to maintain its own police forces to aid the states as and when required to maintain law and order. The central government[16] is currently responsible to maintain seven central police forces across the length and breadth of the country, along with a few other police departments for specialized operations in the fields of intelligence collection, investigation, maintenance of records and providing training. The main objective of the police is to enshrine and monitor the effective implementation of laws at the local and state level, along with ensuring the safety of the citizens. In a populated country like India, the police need to be well-equipped, in terms of the officers, weapons, transportation facilities, etc., so as to they can perform to their full potential. The police officers need to have functional independence to execute duties.

Many police stations have organized women's support groups as well as online chat groups. The support groups run by women are incentivized and aided by the women police stations. In these groups,

[14]https://www.ncbi.nlm.nih.gov/pmc/articles/PMC4216486/#:~:text=Violence%20occurs%20in%20about%2035,data%20from%20Uttar%20Pradesh3.

[15] https://www.india.gov.in/my-government/constitution-india

[16] https://india.unfpa.org/sites/default/files/pub-pdf/435.pdf

psychologists are invited as trainers. By developing a healthy feeling of belongingness, the groups support the sufferers and dismantle the cycle of oppression and hatred. The main aim of the women's groups is to build awareness, empower women and develop strengths so that re-exploitation can be stopped. The policies adopted to strengthen the women police force are well thought and do not suffer from implementational challenges[17]. Gender abuse[18] is prevented by the large-scale educational impact of women police stations' community engagement programmes, which seek to revert the norms that uphold violence against women. The multidisciplinary teams that work in women's police stations are both social order regulators and reform engines. While the findings are encouraging, however, it is difficult to determine how much effect the teams' preventative work with communities has on the local norms that perpetuate gender-based violence.

Need for Women Police Stations in India

The improved representation of women in the administration roles has not only helped women at large to feel empowered, but has also helped reduce crime against them. A gender-diverse administration[19] is essential for creating a safe and secure environment for women. The women often have a different approach to solve the problems as compared to their male counterparts. Women police officers are widely acknowledged as playing an important role in reacting to and combating gender discrimination and crime against women and children. Studies have revealed that domestic violence affects 30 percent of women in the world, and one-third of them suffer physical or sexual violence. Over the last decades, this has been recognized as a grave problem, and international conventions, such as CEDAW (The Convention on Elimination of All Forms of Discrimination Against Women)[20] or Belem do Para (in Brazil)[21], have focused on this issue.

17

https://issuu.com/avocatssansfrontieres/docs/asf_zam_studyantigbvact_2 01708_en

[18] https://ec.europa.eu/info/policies/justice-and-fundamental-rights/gender-equality/gender-based-violence/what-gender-based-violence_en

[19] http://files.eric.ed.gov/fulltext/EJ1210286.pdf

[20] https://www.un.org/womenwatch/daw/cedaw/cedaw.htm

[21] https://www.oas.org/juridico/english/treaties/a-61.html

Several countries are endorsing material measures to reduce domestic violence, ranging from more wide-ranging legislation to introducing several one-stop-centres for women. For example, many Latin American countries have passed new legislative measures to prevent and punish domestic violence between 2005 and 2015: Argentina in 2009, Brazil in 2006, Colombia in 2008, Costa Rica in 2007, El Salvador in 2011, Guatemala in 2008, Mexico in 2007, Nicaragua in 2012, and Venezuela in 2007. In the same decade, Peru, Mexico, Brazil and El Salvador, among others, launched or expanded facilities to provide comprehensive support to victims of domestic violence. One such intervention is women police centres that has been gaining popularity over the last decade. Till now, such police centres have been adopted by Argentina, Bolivia, Ecuador, Ghana, India, Kosovo, Liberia, Nicaragua, Peru, the Philippines, Sierra Leone, South Africa, Uganda and Uruguay. Reports from these countries appear to point out strong effects in some groups of women such as women living in large metropolitan areas and young women aged 15 to 24. Remarkably, the effects are the highest among young women living in metropolitan areas. There are several reasons as to why there is a need for more women police stations in India:

- they empower women and hence increased crime reporting
- women may find it easier and more comfortable to present their incident of crime in front of a woman
- they widen access to justice and reduce corruption
- WPS's have mediation centre to take up matrimonial disputes
- they prevent gender violence as well as crime against women and children

Reports have revealed that the areas with all-woman police stations had a significant increase of 22 in crime reporting. This is due to the reason that women are more comfortable approaching the women police stations. Establishment of women police stations also results in shielding the women victims from the sexual assault by the police officers themselves[22,23].

---

[22]https://services.ecourts.gov.in/ecourtindiaHC/cases/fir1.php?state_cd=16&dist_cd=1&court_code=1&stateNm=Calcutta

[23] https://lawlex.org/lex-bulletin/case-summary-tukaram-and-others-vs-state-of-maharashtra-mathura-rape-case/23555

Need for Gender-Sensitising

Many crimes against women, according to experts, go unreported for a number of reasons, including social stigma and fear of prosecution. A report noted that WPS officers are "more gender-sensitive than other police,[24]" thus, making women feel more at ease approaching them. Hence, setting up of WPS can empower the women and result in increased crime reporting[25].

However, instead of trying to make police work a viable and secure job choice for women, the police departments continue to fail their existing female workers. Sexism and sexual abuse in the police force seem to be widespread across the world. Women police officers themselves become victims of sexual assaults and abuse in police stations which provides a justifiable reason to establish more women police stations in the country. Further, reports have reported the development of a "subculture of oppression"[26] against rape victims. All women police stations, on the other hand, offer a safe space for women.

In the case of *Patel Lila Bhai Ambalal and Etc. vs Patel Kanubhai Mafatlal and Ors. (22 February, 1988)*[27], the Supreme Court observed that in cases of dowry deaths, perpetrators of such crimes often escape the nemesis of the law as a result of inadequate police investigation. The court proposed that a female police officer of appropriate rank and position in the police force be associated with the investigation from the start.

In another case of *Bhagwant Singh vs Commissioner of Police, Delhi (6 May, 1983)*[28], the court recommended, among other things, that a female police officer of appropriate rank and position in the police force be involved with the investigation from the start. It stated, "in situations where the victim's dying declaration can be recorded, it would be more conducive to secure the truth if the victim made the declaration in front of a female police officer who can be expected to inspire

---

[24] http://www.seesac.org/res/files/publication/812.pdf
[25] https://howrahcitypolice.in/women-police-station.html
[26] https://haenfler.sites.grinnell.edu/6549-2/
[27] https://indiankanoon.org/search/?formInput=mafatlal&pagenum=3
[28] https://indiankanoon.org/doc/118375/

trust in the victim". Psychological factors play a role, and their importance cannot be overstated.

Under section 160(1) of CPC (Code of Civil Procedure,1908)[29], women have the right to not being called to the police station. In sexual assault and domestic violence cases, a woman fights both physical injuries and mental trauma. Hence, under this section, women cannot be summoned to the police station or any other location to testify as witnesses. They can only be questioned at their home. During questioning, legal assistance or the assistance of a friend is permitted. However, in the case of *Bilasini Behera vs Unknown (22 December, 2011)*[30], these norms were not followed.

Hence, the establishment of women police stations is a necessary step in mitigating and combating crime in the society against women and children. WPS would provide strength and confidence among women to approach and state their issues for speedy justice. Greater understanding of the administration as well as the consistency of operations would be critical in ensuring that women's perceptions of the process of reporting crimes against them improve.

Conclusion

In a patriarchal society like India, for time immemorial, men have been given the upper hand to stride forward in any leadership roles. It is of utmost importance that women lead the stride from the front, and the department of police offers a vital silver lining. On several occasions, women are afraid to report incidents of crime against them, as they dwell in a state of belief that no action shall be taken, and the culprit might be let loose. There is a certain stigma attached, even today, for the women of the family to go to a police station to report any incident of abuse, where a family member is associated.

All women police stations can send the strongest message in patriarchal environments. According to Sarah Hautzinger[31], "it can be a very effective intervention in areas where women are treated as

---

[29] http://www.bareactslive.com/ACA/ACT379.HTM
[30] https://indiankanoon.org/doc/107672213/
[31] https://www.linkedin.com/in/sarah-hautzinger-a312a777

appendages of male honour."[32]. Women's induction and increased representation in the police force has not only made women feel more confident, but has also helped to reduce crime against them.

In a survey conducted in June 2018, it has been reported that the establishment of all women police stations in India increased the crime reporting by a significant 22 percent. Further, it also led to a 15 percent increase in the women employment in police forces, within a time span of one year from 2015 to 2016.

---

[32] https://www.jstor.org/stable/1409661

19

Transforming Police: Empowerment Issues and Retaining Women Personnel

Anil Bhuimali
Sarmistha Bhattacharya
Sanjib Mandal

Abstract

There is nothing as such a normal day for the police officers, as most of the times they are involved with the critical incidents. Such critical incidents have a significant effect on the police personnel's life.

Women are mostly considered by the society to be unfit in handling the police responsibilities and are always discouraged by the fellow male Police personnel, resulting in affecting the overall image of the police department.

This study intends to identify a few of the issues encountered by women police during their service by extensive literature surveys.

Introduction

The ongoing economic and financial crisis has sparked widespread concern about its effect on development goals[1]. The greater understanding of the present time calls for reform in the systems that oppresses women[2]. It is a fact and known to the common that the success for all has not been uniform[3]. Women have risen to positions of power in some nations, while in others, there are few opportunities

---

[1] Barakso, M. (2004). *Governing NOW: Grassroots activism in the national organization for women.* Cornell University Press.

[2] Leacock, E., Abernethy, V., Bardhan, A., Berndt, C. H., Brown, J. K., Chiñas, B. N., ... & Wadley, S. S. (1978). Women's status in egalitarian society: Implications for social evolution [and comments and reply]. *Current anthropology, 19*(2), 247-275.

[3] Buheji, M. (2018). *Understanding the power of resilience economy: An interdisciplinary perspective to change the world attitude to socio-economic crisis.* Mohamed Buheji.

for them to work or engage in civic affairs and are subjected to significant discriminations.

Need of Empowerment of Women Police

Dominant notions of authority, decision-making and leadership are all constraints faced by the women police officers[4]. It is critical to ensure that women enjoy the rights to which they are entitled not only in the theories or in the debates, but also in the implementation of public policy, legislation and government programmes[5]. Access to work is a relevant issue in levelling opportunities for women[6], with proven programmes promoting women's ability and skills as well as technical and other sectors involving entrepreneurial skills.

The importance of raising awareness through campaigns for fair representation of women in the public sector, leadership training and open hiring practices cannot be overstated[7]. To address the various ongoing issues, society must abolish patriarchal laws and procedures. Only then the personnel of all the genders can be promoted in ensuring the participation at the highest level possible[8]. Many women are now in positions of leadership and decision-making positions too, but at large their skill and authorities are largely affected by non-cooperation of the departmental fellows[9].

Influence of Social and Cultural factors

Owing to the degree of power and discretion granted to police officers, the analysis of police culture is of interest, and it raises the question of how the existence and nature of police culture affect individual

---

[4] Martin, S. E., & Jurik, N. C. (2006). *Doing justice, doing gender: Women in legal and criminal justice occupations*. Sage Publications.
[5] Pruitt, L. J. (2016). *The women in blue helmets: gender, policing, and the un's first all-female peacekeeping unit*. Univ of California Press.
[6] Schechter, S. (1982). *Women and male violence: The visions and struggles of the battered women's movement*. South End Press.
[7] Sinclair, A. (2005). *Doing leadership differently: Gender, power and sexuality in a changing business culture*. Melbourne Univ. Publishing.
[8] Reiner, R. (2010). *The politics of the police*. Oxford University Press.
[9] Strobl, S. (2010). Progressive or neo-traditional? Policewomen in Gulf Cooperation Council (GCC) countries. *Feminist Formations*, 51-74.

officer's working practices[10]. In terms of these two points, the police position is special as the policing duty is unpredictable and unmatched in terms of danger[11] and the amount of power that police officer exercises.

Much work has been done to challenge and analyse the police officers' stereotypical duties. Traditionally, policing has almost considered to be socially segregated[12], resulting in growing of a sense of alienation and unity among the officers[13]. When it comes to women police interactions, the problem of alienation comes up often. If women are not completely included in police culture and working relationships, they can feel alienated, which at large affects the entire department[14] and the female gender per se. When it comes to the tension between the police officers, solidarity arises as a problem[15]. Similarly, the position associated with a stereotypical view of patriarchal system is detrimental to the female officers in discharging their work responsibilities[16].

An accident in which a victim dies, a murder, domestic abuse, theft, and/or rape are all examples of common cases. Involvement in shootings, watching the death of a fellow officer in the line of duty, witnessing a suicide, etc., are among the rare, and are classified as the extreme cases which severely affect the deputed police officers. Several scholars believe that the emphasis on racism has overshadowed the focus on gender parity, resulting in an increase in the discrimination between the male and female police personnel. Indeed, police culture is diverse, and officers themselves take a variety of approaches. There are theoretically a very few professions that are comparable to

---

[10] Chan, J. (1996). Changing police culture. *The British Journal of Criminology*, *36*(1), 109-134.

[11] Westmarland, L. (2008). Police cultures. *Handbook of policing*, *2*, 253-280.

[12] Davis, T. (2007). Gender Inequality In Law Enforcement And Males' Attitudes And Perceptions Toward Women Working In Law Enforcement.

[13] Rumbaut, R. G., & Bittner, E. (1979). Changing conceptions of the police role: A sociological review. *Crime and Justice*, *1*, 239-288.

[14] Perez, A. L., & Strizhko, T. V. (2018). Minority representation, tokenism, and well-being in army units. *Military Psychology*, *30*(5), 449-463.

[15] Punch, M. (2009). *Police corruption: Deviance, accountability and reform in policing*. Routledge.

[16] Skolnick, J. H., & Bayley, D. H. (1988). Theme and variation in community policing. *Crime and justice*, *10*, 1-37.

policing. However, the police culture has been influenced by broader social and political developments and can, therefore, be viewed as a social construct that is not divorced from policing. Policewomen around the world continue to face discrimination and resistance as a result of serving in a male-dominated profession. Gender neutrality theory and practice continue to mask and conceal the underlying gendered substructure, enabling behaviours that perpetuate it to flourish. The police force is profoundly gendered on institutional, cultural and individual levels and cannot be called as a gender-neutral organisation.

Patriarchal Hollow and Women Personnel

Male police officers view women as being physically and mentally incapable of doing the job of policing. Many scholars draw a connection between women's status as non-authoritarian figures in the society and attribute the perceived weakening of police authority to their participation in the policing task[17]. The tendency of male officers to carry out assumed heterosexual stereotypes, such as talking about sexual conquests, harms the spirit of inducting the female officers to the service. Marginalization, alienation, social isolation, sexual and gender abuse characterise women experiences. The women police are forced to maintain the status quo in the male-dominated police force. The principle of disarticulation was not meant to be applied in policing where both female and male police personnel help in the success of the department. The term disarticulation could be used to investigate the perceptions and attitudes of women in their narratives. Disarticulation is a term that can provide some captivating insights into women's possible contribution to a police system that may be oppressive to them.

The Development and Expectations of Society

The women recognise a shift in their identity once they make up their mind to join the police force. However, there is also an important aspect in determining how women want to be seen while discharging their duties. The police service makes a significant change in their life and the way of living. Thereafter, they never intend to look shy or

---

[17] Karlberg, K. (2007). *25 Biggest Mistakes Law Enforcement Officers Make and How to Avoid Them.* Tate Publishing.

anxious, otherwise their official responsibilities are affected. Every woman tries to make it clear that she is a professional who is capable.

It is important to remember that a police officer's work environment and responsibility is not always fixed. The day-to-day personal issues of a women officer also add further tension in their life[18] (including managing finances; saving married life; overcoming domestic violence, health problems, depression, anxiety and anger). Sadly, most of the female police officers encounter these issues during their service career.

Within the police organisation, there seems to have many flawed assumptions. The society largely keeps the expectations from the police officers that they are adequately trained to manage all critical events[19]. It is also believed that officers of the department are well prepared in terms of their ability in handling inquiries[20], and the department offers best practices for its employees, including providing the psychological healing support. Most of the analysis advanced by the scholars suggests that the problems encountered by police organisation are structural and linked to its culture.

Conclusion

No objective analyst can deny the fact that significant progress has been made in a number of key areas by ensuring many efforts to empower women in various sectors to have equitable access to their rights. Many women are now in positions of leadership and decision-making. Hundreds of millions of women are now free of oppression and abuse and have access to education, jobs and participation, owing to the concerted efforts of the governments.

The turning of the emphasis from inequality towards resolving the factors that cause the gender disparities have become more widely recognised. The connection between the gender equality and strong economic growth is becoming clear in every society. There is less

---

[18] Alison, L., & Crego, J. (Eds.). (2012). *Policing critical incidents: Leadership and critical incident management.* Routledge.

[19] Ellison, K. W. (2004). *Stress and the police officer.* Charles C Thomas Publisher.

[20] White, S. O. (1972). A perspective on police professionalization. *Law & Soc'y Rev., 7,* 61.

need felt for special compensatory help for women when both men and women's talent is used in advancing the growth. Women and men must engage and benefit from development through cooperation in order to achieve successful and long-term results.

An organization's success or failure solely depends on the effective management of the employees' needs. By identifying the role of the department and being actively involved in the planning, preparation[21] and implementation of mental health programmes that meet the needs of its employees, policing can deliver its best service to the society[22].

---

[21] Bayley, D. H. (1994). *Police for the Future*. Oxford University Press on Demand.
[22] More, H. W., & Miller, L. S. (2014). *Effective police supervision*. Routledge.

9 781922 617071